NATURAL for Arthritis

MW00366903

The Best Alternative Methods for Relieving Pain and Stiffness

from
Food & Herbs
to
Acupuncture & Homeopathy

GLENN S. ROTHFELD, M.D.

AND SUZANNE LeVERT

Rodale Press, Inc.
Emmaus, Pennsylvania

This book is intended as a reference volume only, not as a medical manual. The information given here is designed to help you make informed decisions about your health. It is not intended as a substitute for any treatment that may have been prescribed by your doctor. If you suspect that you have a medical problem, we urge you to seek competent medical help.

Library of Congress Cataloging-in-Publication Data

Rothfeld, Glenn.
    Natural medicine for arthritis : the best alternative methods for
relieving pain and stiffness / Glenn S. Rothfeld and Suzanne LeVert.
      p.   cm.
    Includes index.
    ISBN 0–87596–287–4 paperback
     1. Arthritis—Alternate treatment. I. LeVert, Suzanne. II Title.
RC933.R6677   1996
516.7'2206—dc20   95–13305

Distributed in the book trade by St. Martin's Press

4 6 8 10 9 7 5 3   paperback

—————— OUR MISSION ——————

We publish books that empower people's lives.

——— RODALE BOOKS ———

Dedication

....

To Magi for her continued love and partnership.

To my parents,
Daniel and Eleanor Rothfeld, for their
encouragement and support.
G. S. R.

Acknowledgments

....

I would like to thank Madeleine Morel, Barbara
Lowenstein, and Rodale Press for their help in hatching
and shepherding this idea; AMR'TA, makers of IBIS,
an extraordinary data base of natural medicine;
Ben Benjamins, Catherine LeBlanc, Dr. Daren Fan,
Dr. Richard Glickman-Simon, Lori Grace,
Nancy Lipman, and others who helped me with their
comments and encouragement. I am also grateful
to the many patients who brought me ideas and inspired
me with their own journeys toward better health.

Contents

"Nature heals under the auspices of the medical profession."

Haven Emerson

Arthritis and
Alternative Medicine

$\mathcal{I}$n the United States today, more than 15 percent of the entire population—or about 40 million people—suffer from arthritis. It is a disease that does not discriminate; men and women of all races are at risk of developing some form of arthritis, and close to 200,000 children suffer from its effects. This disease, of which there are more than 100 different forms, involves the inflammation of joints, surrounding tendons, ligaments, and cartilage, as well as destruction of bone. It can affect any part of the body, from the feet to the knees, back, shoulders, elbows, fingers and, in certain types of arthritis, heart, lung, or other organs as well.

The symptoms of arthritis range from mild aches and flulike discomfort to all-consuming, crippling, chronic pain. Currently, no cure exists for arthritis. Instead, it is a chronic condition that continues to perplex and frustrate both those who suffer with it and their healers. In this book, we will introduce you to several different theories about the disease and what they mean to the person who has it, as well as outline in detail some effective treatment strategies—all from a holistic, alternative medicine perspective.

Humankind has suffered from arthritis for as long as we've been recording medical history. X-ray studies of bones from our earliest ancestors, including mummified Egyptians, attest that arthritis has long been a significant health problem. The credit for first describing the condition goes to the Greek physician Hippocrates, who gave it the Greek word for "swollen joint." Rheumatism, a word that we still often use interchangeably with arthritis, derives from the Greek word *rheumatismos*, which means "flowing mucus," referring to the swelling that occurs when fluid fills a joint. Some historical sources estimate that as much as 70 percent of the population of ancient Rome had some form of arthritis, a fact that led researchers to postulate that the Romans used their infamously decadent "Roman baths" as therapy for this often painful and limiting disease.

Chances are that you or someone you love suffers with arthritis to one degree or another. Like so many of your contemporaries, you are looking for a safe way to alleviate its symptoms and stop (or at least slow down) its often cruel progression. Unfortunately, we've been brought up to assume that all things medical can be quickly resolved with drugs and/or surgery. We remain stubbornly (and, in the end, counterproductively) distanced from the intricate nature and quality of health. We need to better recognize the work that it takes, on both the patient's and the healer's parts, to return to that precious state.

The Challenge of Chronic Disease

Within the modern, Western medical tradition, physicians and researchers often divide health problems into those considered *acute* and those considered *chronic*. Acute health problems generally begin abruptly with a single, readily identifiable cause. Scientific literature has thoroughly documented the course of these illnesses, which tend to respond well to specific treatments, such as medication or surgery. When treatment succeeds in eliminating the symptoms and effects of the acute illness, doctors consider patients "cured"—brought back to a normal state of health.

Appendicitis is an example of an acute illness. So is an infection with the bacterium *Streptococcus*, such as tonsillitis. Each has distinct symptoms: nausea and abdominal pain in the case of appendicitis; sore throat with swollen tonsils and fever with tonsillitis. Appendicitis necessitates surgery followed by a period of recovery. Tonsillitis usually resolves quickly with a 10-day course of antibiotic medication, usually consisting of penicillin.

Chronic illnesses, on the other hand, tend to start slowly, proceed slowly, and last over several years, even over an entire lifespan. Doctors usually have trouble diagnosing a chronic illness since its symptoms and course tend to be subtle (at least at first) and unpredictable. Unlike acute disease, chronic disease often has several possible, sometimes coexisting causes, ranging from genetic factors to lifestyle and environmental influences to individual physiological qualities. Almost by definition, chronic illnesses have no "cure," no simple solution. Because each of them generally has more than one cause, no one drug or surgical procedure is able to remedy them.

As different as each type of chronic illness may be from another— asthma, for instance, has a set of symptoms and effects markedly different from arthritis—they have a number of disturbing similarities. Indeed, the lives of all those with chronic illnesses almost inevitably change, both physically and emotionally. Without proper care and patient involvement in an effective therapy program, those with a chronic illness like arthritis often must curtail physical activities such as grocery shopping, knitting, golfing, and gardening. As a result, muscles and tendons become weak from lack of use. Should such limitations persist, a sense of isolation and helplessness begins to sink in, leaving the person with a chronic illness vulnerable to clinical depression.

As you'll see in Chapter 2, modern mainstream medicine offers few successful options for the treatment of arthritis. It remains stymied by the complexity of the disease and, perhaps most important, by its apparently systemic and fundamental nature. Holistic medicine, on the other hand, is remarkably suited to exploring just these issues. Its view of health is based on establishing and maintaining internal balance, of helping the body to maintain its own proper structure and function by providing it with all the nutrients, physical exercise, and emotional support it requires. Here are just a few of the issues you may want to consider while thinking about holistic medicine:

Holistic Medicine

Involves few side effects compared with pharmacology or surgery. Alternative medicine works by helping the body to heal itself. Drugs, on the other hand, including those used to alleviate the pain and inflammation of arthritis, work either by taking over the body's functions or by masking the pain that might otherwise help the body protect itself against further harm. The body never fully heals, then, but is compelled to operate despite the problems. Moreover, drugs often have side effects—such as drowsiness and confusion (common to many painkillers) or gastric problems (stemming from aspirin use)—that alternative therapies generally avoid.

Focuses on the individual, not the condition. Practitioners of natural medicine recognize that every person with arthritis develops the disease under a different set of circumstances; and because there are so many different causes of arthritis, no one type of therapy will cure it. Treating arthritis with alternative medicine involves not a simple prescription or operation, but a comprehensive plan that recognizes your unique emotional, spiritual, and physical makeup.

Involves the whole body. According to most alternative disciplines, the joints, tendons, and cartilage involved in the arthritis process do not exist in isolation from the rest of the body. Nor do they remain unaffected by emotions, thoughts, or external stressors. While the average rheumatologist concentrates on the particular joints affected by arthritis, the Chinese practitioner, chiropracter, or herbalist looks at the whole person from head to toe, physically and emotionally.

Validates the emotional component of health. Although it seems clear that external stresses and/or emotional upheavals have a direct impact on the body's ability to function, Western medicine has resisted using this knowledge to prevent or treat disease. Natural medicine acknowledges the integral role our emotions play in maintaining health, and its traditions have used this knowledge in creating a comprehensive treatment plan for virtually every disease and condition. As you'll discover by reading this book, arthritis is no exception. The more relaxed you are, the more manageable your symptoms will be.

Prevents as well as treats. Maintaining the body's natural, balanced state is the goal of natural medicine. If you visit a homeopath for treatment of your arthritis, for instance, you may find that you no longer suffer as many colds or flus or that the treatment alleviates another recurrent health problem as well. This is because the remedies applied work on many different levels and systems throughout the body.

Helps you find the natural rhythm of health. Your body is a remarkable vessel of biochemical actions and reactions that allow you to breathe, to digest your food, to dream, and to hope. Natural approaches to health and healing allow your body to work as nature intended, without the need for artificial and potentially side effect–ridden interventions.

For the reasons outlined above, you may decide to join the millions of Americans who have turned to alternative therapies to treat their arthritis or other conditions. This book is intended to help you sort through the many alternative approaches available and decide which ones may work best for your particular situation. You or someone you love is looking for help. The pain, swelling, and stiffness of arthritis have made life more difficult and unmanageable, and you may fear what the future holds if you do not find an effective therapy. In this book, you'll learn the basics of several alternative options, one or more of which may hold an answer for you.

Nine Natural Approaches
to Treating Arthritis

Before we outline the various approaches covered in this book, we must stress—and we'll reiterate this point later—how important it is for you to visit a mainstream physician for an evaluation of your condition. By taking advantage of mainstream diagnostic procedures, you'll be able to rule out serious medical problems such as tumors, infections, and structural problems that may be at the root of your condition—and may require a more immediate mainstream treatment to resolve.

On the other hand, if you're like most people with arthritis, you've already discovered the limitations of modern medicine when it comes to treating your condition. The good news is that you may well hold the solution within yourself: Your own body can heal itself if given the right ingredients and the right environment.

Outlined below are nine different alternative methods. The first three—diet, exercise, and meditation—you can do on your own. Except for obtaining permission from a physician or practitioner to start a new exercise program, these are changes you can make by yourself. The other six techniques involve philosophies and techniques that, generally speaking, stem from very different systems of thought. We'll introduce you to their basic theories and therapies in hopes that, should one or more of them interest you, you'll take the time to explore them more thoroughly by reading other books and visiting qualified practitioners.

THE FOOD LINK

Chapter Four discusses the connection between what you eat and how you feel, specifically the impact of food allergies on destructive joint inflammation. We outline the principles of finding and treating food reactions and include specific food recommendations known to help prevent arthritis flare-ups or alleviate the pain once it has begun. Furthermore, we provide a list of the nutritional supplements known to affect the arthritis process, including vitamin B_6, vitamin C, calcium, and magnesium, among others.

EXERCISE AND REST

Your body needs to move in order for you to stay well. Your brain, your heart, your internal organs, your muscles—they all need the increased blood flow and stimulation that exercise provides. For your joints, this statement of fact holds special meaning. By moving your joints daily, you help keep them fully mobile. You also strengthen surrounding muscles, which means providing joints with extra support. Weight-bearing exercise helps keep your bones strong and helps reduce your chance of osteoporosis, a disease of thinning bones often associated with arthritis. Moving your joints also helps to transport nutrients and waste products to and from your cartilage—the body tissue that protects the ends of your bones. In Chapter 5, we'll show you some of the best exercises for you, depending on what part of your body arthritis affects. We'll also outline a general fitness program designed to condition your whole body safely and effectively, which will both help keep you healthy and improve your general outlook.

MEDITATION AND RELAXATION

Chapter 6 describes the relationship between stress and chronic pain of any kind, including that related to arthritis. There we will guide you through several methods of meditation and relaxation designed to help you recognize and then release your own particular brand of negative stress. These methods include progressive relaxation, visualization, and biofeedback, among others.

ACUPUNCTURE AND CHINESE MEDICINE

Stemming from a centuries-old tradition, Chinese medicine and acupuncture view health not only as the absence of disease, but also as the existence of a balanced and harmonious internal environment. Humanity is seen as part of a larger creation—the universe itself—and is thus subject to the same laws that govern the stars, the soil, and the sea. Chapter 7 explains this unique philosophy and its relevance to arthritis, as well as outlines the techniques of acupuncture, Chinese herbal medicine, and the exercise system known as qi-gong as they relate to the treatment of arthritis.

AYURVEDA: MEDICINE FROM INDIA

Based on a system developed in India around the fifth century B.C., Ayurveda, like Chinese medicine, considers health within a universal context. Within the human body, universal forces exist as an energy or life force called *prana*. Prana provides every human being with the vitality and endurance to live in harmony with the universe, as well as offers the body the power to heal itself. In Chapter 8, you'll see how an Ayurvedic practitioner might consider your condition and discover how your arthritis might be treated according to Ayurvedic principles. Such treatment may include yoga, herbal remedies, and meditation exercises. In addition, certain dietary recommendations may be made.

CHIROPRACTIC AND OSTEOPATHY

Chapter 9 introduces you to two related branches of alternative medicine: chiropractic and osteopathy. According to the theory behind chiropractic therapy, the spine is the well from which the body's innate intelligence springs. If the vertebrae are not properly aligned, this intelligence cannot flow to other parts of the body to assure their proper functioning. Realigning the spine can thus alleviate arthritic pain, and may even work to resolve the underlying causes of the disorder.

Osteopathy is another system that involves adjusting the body in order to improve its overall function and health. Osteopaths receive standard physician training (their degree, doctor of osteopathy, is equivalent to a medical doctor), but their education also includes courses on how to adjust the spine and other skeletal structures in order to relieve pain and improve motion and circulation.

HEALING TOUCH: BODYWORK AND MASSAGE

In Chapter 10, you'll read about several different movement awareness and massage therapies, such as the Alexander technique and Rolfing, all of which attempt both to alleviate current pain and realign the body to help reduce the pain of future arthritis flare-ups. Some of these techniques require the involvement of a trained professional; others you can learn to do on your own with some guidance. In either case, you're bound to find massage to be a powerful healing tool.

THE POWER OF HERBS

Herbal medicine and its cousin aromatherapy use plants, herbs, and other natural substances—including venom extracted from honeybees—to stimulate the body to return to the state of internal balance we call health. Though herbs are medicines, they tend to be much safer than chemical drugs for a variety of reasons: they are less potent, more recognizable to the body as natural substances, and usually used in combinations and potencies that minimize side effects. Derived from plants, each oil has its own distinct odor that stimulates an array of emotional and psychological responses. Chapter 11 discusses how you can use herbs and oils to treat your case of arthritis.

LIKE CURES LIKE: HOMEOPATHY

Chapter 12 explores homeopathy and its relationship to arthritis. A system of medicine that attempts to harness the body's own healing power to fight disease and maintain health, homeopathy was developed by a nineteenth-century German scientist named Samuel Hahnemann. It is based on the principle that "like cures like," that medications should be given not to counteract the symptoms of illness, as they are in mainstream medicine, but rather to stimulate the body to cure itself. Because arthritis involves the swelling and tenderness of inflammation, homeopathic remedies for arthritis tend to concentrate on helping the body to reverse this process.

Following these chapters on the basics of alternative medicine, Chapter 13 raises and answers some of the most common questions about arthritis and the various therapies offered here to treat it. Then, in *Natural Resources*, page 168, we provide you with a host of resources, including organizations, associations, and books, that will guide you should you choose to further explore any or all of the methods outlined here.

In the meantime, however, we feel it's important for you to gain an understanding of what arthritis is on a strictly anatomical and physiological level. Chapter 2 will explain exactly what happens to the joints and tissues of the body when the disease of arthritis takes hold.

"It is more important to know what kind of patient has a disease than what kind of disease a patient has."

Hippocrates

A Medical Overview

*E*very 33 seconds—more than a million times a year—another American develops arthritis. Today, the Arthritis Foundation estimates that 40 million Americans, or one in seven, have some form of arthritis. Because arthritis tends to affect older people more often than younger people, that number is almost certain to increase in the coming years as our population in general begins to age. Current statistics indicate that the number of Americans ages 65 and older will double between 1990 and 2040.

In addition to the personal toll arthritis exacts, a tall financial bill results as well. Arthritis and related disorders cost the nation more than $50 billion every year in lost wages, medical bills, and other expenses. The National Arthritis Workgroup of the National Institutes of Health estimates that the disorders will add more than $95 billion to the nation's annual health costs by the year 2000. As it is, arthritis already accounts for an annual total of at least 26 million lost workdays and another 500 million restricted workdays every year.

What causes the disease at the root of this enormous health care problem? Who is at risk for developing it? Are there ways to prevent it? To cure it? These are the questions motivating medical researchers in laboratories around the world. If you or someone in your family suffers from arthritis, they are questions that demand an answer without delay.

Understanding Arthritis

The human skeleton, made up of more than 200 bones, is strong, resilient, and equipped with certain structures, called joints, that allow the body to bend, twist, and move in all the human ways to which we are accustomed. The joints of our fingers permit us to pick up utensils, to write with a pencil, and to grip a toothbrush, a golf club, or a knitting needle. Our knees bend so that we can run, kneel, and climb endless flights of stairs. Our hips pivot, making it possible for us to dance, crouch in the garden, and curl up to sleep. All of these joints as well as those of our elbows, spine, toes, and ankles allow us to perform the very movements that make us vital, active people.

As is so often true, however, we tend not to appreciate how remarkable the human body is until it begins to fail us. Most cases of arthritis begin slowly, bit by bit robbing an individual of a touch of mobility here, a moment of comfort there. Often, however, the disease progresses, eating into daily activities and imposing ever deepening levels and periods of pain. To fully understand this process, it is necessary to first examine a healthy joint and how it behaves.

THE ANATOMY OF A JOINT

Simply put, a joint is the point of intersection of two or more bones. We further characterize joints in a number of different ways. First, joints are characterized by the *degree of motion* they allow, from very subtle to free range of movement. The skull, for instance, contains joints along suture lines which allow very tiny movement in one direction. The joints in the hips, wrist, and ankles, in contrast, allow pretty free movement—up and down, sideways, and even a circular motion. Thus, free-moving joints are further categorized by the *direction in which they move*. Here are some of the major categories of free-moving joints and how they work:

Ball-and-Socket Joint. In this type of joint, the end of one bone is round and fits neatly into a cuplike socket that forms the end of another bone. Such a construction permits movement in all directions. The hip and shoulder are two examples of ball-and-socket joints.

Gliding Joint. A gliding joint is constructed in such a way as to allow for only limited, gliding movement; the ligaments and other tissues around each gliding joint limit motion. The vertebrae and the ribs are examples of gliding joints.

Hinge Joint. This type of joint permits extensive movement—but only in one direction. Elbow joints, knee joints, and the joints of the fingers are all examples of hinge joints.

Saddle Joint. So named because the opposing bones are convex and concave and fit together to form what looks like a rider upon a saddle, this type of joint can move up and down and side to side, but cannot rotate. The wrist and thumb are two examples of saddle joints.

Finally, we also refer to joints as being either *weight-bearing* or *nonweight-bearing*, depending on their function in the body. Weight-bearing joints, such as the ankles, knees, hips, and vertebrae, bear the brunt of the physical stress placed on the body. Joints in the upper body, such as the fingers, wrists, and shoulders, are considered non-weight-bearing joints.

As different in function as joints tend to be, all free-moving joints—such as those described above and the ones most commonly involved in arthritis—have similar components that, if healthy, allow movement to occur without pain or inflammation. Let's examine them one by one, then explore what happens when arthritis takes hold:

Cartilage. Cartilage is a smooth, resilient material that coats the ends of bones, forming a cushion that protects the bones from rubbing against each other. Cartilage has a slick exterior, which allows bones to slide over each other, and a spongy, compressible interior that is able to absorb shock. It is composed mostly of water and a substance called *collagen* (made up of long protein molecules woven together). Collagen also forms the connective tissue that makes up the white, inelastic fibers of the ligaments and bones.

Joint Capsule. Also called the synovial sac, the joint capsule completely encases the ends of bones and cartilage. Lining the joint capsule is the *synovial membrane*, a thin, delicate lining rich in blood vessels and nerve endings. In a healthy joint, this membrane produces a clear, viscous fluid that acts to lubricate the joint and nourish the cartilage, which has no blood supply of its own.

Connective Tissues. Thick, cordlike fibers called *ligaments*, anchored to the bone on either side of the joint, help form the outside of the joint capsule. Ligaments help to keep the bones in correct alignment. Strong fibrous bands called *tendons* attach *muscles* to bones. Muscles are tissues made up of fibers that are able to contract, allowing the parts and organs of the body to move.

Bursae. Just outside the joint capsule lie small fluid-filled sacs called bursae. Bursae produce a lubricating liquid that helps muscles, tendons, and bones slide over one another.

When all of these components work together as they should, the human body is able to move smoothly and with remarkable flexibility and grace.

The Process of Arthritis: Causes and Risk Factors

As discussed in Chapter 1, arthritis is a term used to describe a group of diseases that affect one or more of the structures in and around the joint, including the synovial membranes, cartilage, muscles, tendons, ligaments, muscles, bones, and/or bursae. In medicine, the suffix -*itis* means inflammation. Inflammation is actually the immune system's response to infection or injury. Most forms of arthritis involve this immune system reaction. Following is a discussion of some of the most common categories of arthritis according to the structures that are most involved:

Joint Membrane Inflammation. This type of arthritis involves inflammation of the synovial membrane, the thin lining of the joint. When this occurs, the normally smooth, thin, inner membrane becomes thickened and swollen. Both the joint fluid and the synovial lining become inundated with white blood cells—cells of the immune system produced when injury or infection occurs. In addition to the pain this process causes, the white blood cells may also produce substances that can wear away the bone's protective cartilage to form gaps called erosions. Eventually, if the condition goes untreated, so much cartilage can wear away that the ends of the bones become exposed and rub together. Eventually bone erosion and destruction may also occur. Also called *synovitis,* these processes are the hallmarks of *rheumatoid arthritis,* the second most common form of arthritis (after osteoarthritis).

Cartilage Breakdown. Degeneration of cartilage, the material that covers the ends of bones, is a major characteristic of *osteoarthritis*. When cartilage breaks down, it becomes cracked and uneven, exposing the bones and allowing them to rub against each other. The bones may then thicken, cysts (pockets of fluid) may form, and joint space may narrow further. A degenerative joint disease most associated with aging or a previous injury to the joint, osteoarthritis may or may not involve inflammation as part of its process.

Metabolic Disorders. In this type of arthritis, tiny crystals form in the joint space when the level of certain blood chemicals becomes too high. White blood cells rush to the site, causing the joint to become inflamed and painful. *Gout* is the most common form of this type of arthritis and occurs when too much uric acid, a blood protein, is present in the body.

Infections. A number of infectious agents, including viruses and bacteria, can invade the joint spaces, resulting in inflammation. The most common types of infectious arthritis are acute and caused by bacteria, particularly the *gonococcus* (which causes gonorrhea) and *staphylococcus* (which causes several different types of disease). A recently identified type of chronic infectious arthritis is called *Lyme disease*, named after the town in Connecticut that reported the first cases. Caused by an organism called a spirochete, Lyme disease is transmitted to humans through the deer tick. Its symptoms range from transitory flulike symptoms to severe, persistent joint pain. Generally speaking, however, acute infectious arthritis is not a common disease, and most cases occur in people who have preexisting arthritis or a disease (such as cancer) that lowers their immune response to these invading organisms.

Traumas and Injuries. Over time, undue stress placed on the joints can result in inflammation of the tendons and muscles, as well as the joint capsule, causing pain and stiffness. Damage to knees caused by the stress that being overweight places on these joints is one example of trauma-induced arthritis; bone changes in the feet of runners and basketball players is another.

Connective Tissue Disorders. Connective tissue diseases involve inflammation of tissues that support and connect tissues and body organs. Connective tissue is the major component of bone, cartilage, skin, and blood vessles. A systemic arthritis, such as *rheumatoid arthritis* or *systemic lupus erythematosus*, often affects connective tissues throughout the body, causing achiness and fever in addition to local joint inflammation. Sometimes, these diseases can cause damage to other body organs as well.

Spinal Stiffening. In a form of arthritis known as *ankylosing spondylitis,* the ligaments and tendons attached to the vertebrae become inflamed, thickened, and scarred. The bones in these joints may grow into one another, eventually becoming fused, resulting in stiffness and loss of mobility. Ankylosing spondylitis is often related to other disorders, such as Reiter's syndrome (characterized by urinary, eye, and joint inflammation) or ulcerative colitis (a chronic inflammatory disease of the large intestine and rectum).

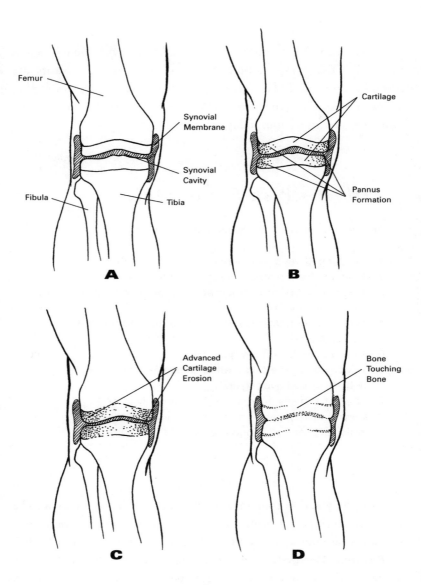

Rheumatoid Arthritis

Rheumatoid arthritis is a degenerative condition. It begins with inflammation of the synovial membrane (a) and progresses to the erosion of cartilage (b and c). Eventually, the joint cavity is destroyed, the bones rub together and erode, and the joint may be fused (d).

As you can see, several things can go wrong with the joints and surrounding tissues in your body. Still mysterious, even to doctors, are the reasons why such damage occurs. Are you at risk for developing one or more of these conditions? Take the self-test below to see how arthritis might affect you, today or in the future:

Arthritis Risk Factor Quiz

Answer yes or no to the following questions:

1. Have you always maintained a healthy weight?
2. Does any form of arthritis run in the family?
3. Have you sustained a traumatic or repetitive strain injury to any of your joints?
4. Have you been diagnosed with an autoimmune disease, such as lupus?
5. Do you exercise on a regular basis?
6. Do you eat a varied diet rather than a few of the same foods over and over again?
7. Do you have any allergies or food sensitivities?
8. Are you taking any medications on a regular basis, particulary for high blood pressure?

How did you do? Your answers may indicate that you may well be at risk for developing arthritis or for making a minor condition worse. Let's see what your answers might mean to the future of your health.

Excess Weight. The most common form of arthritis is osteoarthritis, a condition that can be triggered or exacerbated by the added stress and strain to the joints caused by carrying too much weight. When someone with osteoarthritis or, in fact, any type of arthritis, is overweight, he or she places an additional burden on joints already made vulnerable by disease. Maintaining a healthy weight, therefore, can help you to both prevent the onset of arthritis and limit the number and intensity of flare-ups if you already suffer from the disease.

Heredity. It has long been observed that arthritis tends to run in families. That is, if your parents, grandparents, or siblings suffer from one type of arthritis, you may have a greater risk of developing the disease than someone without a family history. Indeed, genetics—the study of the principles and mechanics of heredity—may well provide the biggest clue to the mystery of arthritis so far uncovered. Several years ago, scientists discovered that some common arthritic diseases are associated with the presence of certain genetic markers known as human leukocyte antigens (HLAs). Most people with rheumatoid arthritis, for example, carry the genetic marker HLA-DR4, while those with ankylosing spondylitis carry HLA-B27. The presence of these markers may indicate that the affected individual has a greater risk of developing arthritis than someone without the marker.

However, it must be stressed that having a family history of arthritis or even having one of the genetic markers that indicate a predisposition to the disease, does not mean that you are doomed to develop it. In fact, researchers believe that genetics and some other trigger—such as an infection, allergy, injury, exposure to chemicals, or an autoimmune response—must work together in order to stimulate the arthritic process. Avoiding or limiting your exposure to these triggers may well prevent you from developing arthritis, no matter how strong your family history of arthritis is.

Trauma and Injury. Several different types of arthritis appear to be triggered or exacerbated by trauma or injury, either to the joint itself or to the surrounding ligaments, bursae, muscles, and tendons. Worth special mention are repetitive strain injuries, caused by performing the same movement over and over again, such as typing at a computer console or lifting heavy packages on a loading dock. Over time, such injuries may cause constant low-grade inflammatory reactions that end up permanently damaging joints.

Infections. Infectious arthritis occurs as a complication of a disease caused by a virus, bacterium, fungus, or other agent. In most cases, it results in a case of acute arthritis that dissipates once the infection is treated. Among the most common infectious triggers are the sexually transmitted chlamydial disease and gonorrhea, as well as *Salmonella* and *Shigella*, two bacteria known to cause gastrointestinal disorders. As far as chronic arthritis goes, the most common infectious trigger is Lyme disease, carried by deer ticks. Protecting yourself from exposure to these infectious agents is one way to help cut down your risk of developing arthritis or avoid flare-ups should you already have the disease.

Exercise. Exercise—perhaps the single most important factor in maintaining the health of our joints, bones, and supporting structures— is often the most neglected aspect of our daily lives. As well as helping the heart, brain, and other internal organs stay healthy and fit, exercise has special advantages as far as the joints are concerned. By moving your joints daily, you'll keep them fully mobile and supple. Joint movement also helps to transport essential nutrients and waste products to and from your cartilage. Weight-bearing exercises help to strengthen your muscles, providing your joints with extra support, as well as help to reduce your chances of developing osteoporosis, a disease characterized by thinning bones and often associated with arthritis.

Varied Diet. Food allergies and sensitivities may be more common than we realize. By eating a varied diet, rich with vitamins and minerals, you'll stand a greater chance of providing your body with all the raw ingredients it needs to be healthy. If your diet is deficient in one or more essential nutrients, however, you may be putting your joints at risk for deterioration and pain. In addition, eating too much sugar, drinking too much alcohol, and consuming too much caffeine may also have an impact on the health of your joints and your body in general.

Allergies or Food Sensitivities. The link between allergies, particularly those caused by the foods we eat, and arthritis remains the subject of intense investigation by scientists around the world. Allergies result from an overstimulated immune system, the same body system implicated in the process of arthritis. If you suffer from allergies, then you may be at increased risk of developing arthritis or of provoking flare-ups should you already have the disease. Furthermore, you may be eating foods that, unbeknownst to you, exacerbate your condition. Foods of the nightshade family, such as eggplant and tomatoes, are among those most closely linked to arthritis.

Medications. In rare cases, it appears that some medications may trigger the onset of certain arthritic diseases, including systemic lupus erythematosus and gout. In most cases, the arthritic symptoms disappear once the person stops taking the offending medication. If you take any of the following medications and suffer from symptoms of arthritis, check with your doctor to make sure you are not experiencing a drug reaction:

> *Isoniazid* and *ethambutol* (used to treat tuberculosis)
> *Hydralazine* (used to treat high blood pressure)
> *Procainamide* (for heart rhythm problems)
> *Chlorpromazine* (used for a variety of problems, including migraine headache and nausea)
> *Aspirin* (if taken on a regular basis, may cause buildup of uric acid, leading to gout)

Diagnosing Arthritis

As you can see, the causes and courses of arthritis are varied and often hard to pinpoint. In some cases, the aches and pains we feel will never receive a definitive diagnosis at all, but will be labeled "arthritis" or "rheumatism" simply because no other conclusion can be reached.

If that's the case, you may ask, why bother to see a doctor at all? Without alarming you unduly, there are some serious medical problems that have chronic joint pain as one of their symptoms, including viral and bacterial infections and certain cancers. Ruling out these conditions, as well as pinpointing exactly which joints are currently involved in the arthritic process and to what degree, are among the reasons you should see your physician if you experience joint pain.

If you're like most people, your primary care physician will be the first to consider your symptoms. Because arthritis is such a common condition, he may be experienced enough to make an accurate initial diagnosis. Depending on the severity of the disease and the level of his expertise, he may then refer you to a *rheumatologist*, a specialist fully trained in general internal medicine who has studied arthritic diseases an additional two or three years. Another specialist you may consult, especially if your problem is injury-related, is an *orthopedist*. An orthopedist is a surgical specialist in the treatment of joints, muscles, and related structures. Should your doctor suspect that nerve damage has occurred, he may refer you to a *neurologist*, a specialist in the study and treatment of diseases of the central and peripheral nervous system. If you also have rashes and other skin problems, as is often the case with lupus, you may decide to see a *dermatologist*, a doctor specializing in the skin.

Internal medicine, rheumatology, orthopedics, neurology, dermatology—the list of specialities involved in the treatment of arthritis seems daunting. In fact, this highlights a crucial aspect of disease as viewed by mainstream, Western medicine. According to this perspective, each part of the body is considered a distinct and separate entity, largely unconnected to the others. Alternative medicine, on the other hand, views the body as an integrated whole: To distinguish between a problem that causes a rash and a problem that causes joint pain—simply because two different areas of the body are involved—is considered an arbitrary and meaningless procedure within this tradition. Furthermore, and perhaps even more fundamentally, alternative medicine does not, as so often does mainstream medicine, make a sharp distinction between the physical and emotional. An alternative medical practitioner is likely to view the state of your mental and emotional health as equal in importance to the state of your physical being. In fact, you may be surprised at how much time you spend discussing personal issues and habits with an alternative practitioner.

Despite what might be considered shortcomings in the mainstream approach to a chronic condition like arthritis, modern medicine does offer the best technological tools for making a diagnosis—at least from a purely mechanical perspective. When you visit your doctor for an evaluation, you will probably be taken through an exam consisting of some or all of the following:

Taking a Medical History

The first step in almost every medical exam—mainstream or alternative—consists of the physician or practitioner asking you several questions about your current medical condition, your past experiences, and your family history of disease. He will also delve into aspects of your lifestyle—what kind of work you do, your hobbies, the amount of stress under which you live, and what kind of diet you consume on a regular basis, among other issues—at least to some degree. Generally speaking, an alternative practitioner will pay far more attention to these matters than will a mainstream physician.

Of special importance is a thorough and accurate description of your joint pain and other symptoms. Your doctor is likely to ask you some or all of the questions listed below. Before your first appointment, take a look at these questions and think about how you'll answer them. The more accurate you can be about your symptoms and what you think may contribute to them, the closer your doctor can get to a realistic diagnosis and treatment plan.

Things to Think About
Before You See Your Doctor

1. Which of your joints hurt?
2. When is the first time you remember having pain? Did it follow an injury or trauma?
3. Has the joint pain spread to more than one joint?
4. Is the pain sharp or dull?
5. What makes the pain get worse?
6. What makes the pain go away?
7. What time of day is the pain at its worst?
8. Do your joints lock or give way?
9. Do you feel stiff in the morning?
10. Do you have fever? Have you noticed a rash?

11. Have you lost or gained weight?
12. What past medical treatment have you had, for this problem and for others?
13. Are you currently taking drugs (either prescription medication or illegal substances)?
14. Does your arthritis affect your ability to work?
15. Do you feel unusally tired during the day?
16. Do you have symptoms of depression (listlessness, sadness, helplessness, loss of appetite) or anxiety?

After you and your doctor sort through these issues and discuss all aspects of your past medical history, you will likely embark upon the second part of the evaluation procedure: the physical examination.

THE PHYSICAL EXAM: WHAT TO EXPECT

As you might suspect, the doctor will want to take a careful look at the way you move in general, the way your joints react to specific movements, and how much pain these movements cause you. Your physician will probably begin her evaluation by systematically examining all of your joints on both sides of your body. Most likely, she will start with your hands, since the hands are involved in many different types of arthritic conditions. As the doctor touches your joints, she will be looking for signs of inflammation, including redness, swelling, and/or tenderness, especially of the synovial membrane (joint lining). Synovial inflammation may also cause the joint to become thickened and rubbery, a state that the doctor can feel by pressing gently on the affected joint.

The doctor will also pay careful attention to your hips, knees, spine, and specifically any joints that have caused you the most trouble in the past. She may ask you to perform certain movements, like bending down to touch your toes or taking deep breaths to see how flexible your spine is. Because joints can lose function as a result of severe inflammation or cartilage degeneration, your doctor will need to assess the range of motion of your joints. Range of motion is usually measured in degrees. The knee joint, for example, can normally be extended to a straight line, or 180 degrees. If the knee is damaged, the doctor may describe the problem as a 30-degree lack of extension.

Some forms of arthritis produce easily recognized signs of illness, some of which are permanent and others reversible. Lupus, for example, often involves a characteristic facial skin rash as well as a related blood vessel problem (known as Raynaud's syndrome) that results in fingers turning blue and white in the cold. Rheumatoid arthritis can produce characteristic changes in the shapes of the fingers, which may become crooked or drift to the side. Osteoarthritis may produce knobby enlargements in the joint of the fingertips—called Heberden's nodes—which may appear in one or more fingers of an afflicted individual. By assessing such changes, and other accompanying symptoms, your doctor can further define your medical condition.

Finally, depending on the conclusions your doctor reaches from your medical history and physical exam, he or she may suggest you undergo one or more of the following *laboratory tests*. Generally speaking, however, only a few tests should be necesary in order to confirm the doctor's preliminary diagnosis.

BLOOD TESTS

Complete Blood Count. Because inflammation can cause certain typical changes in a person's blood count, this blood test is often performed to see if the levels of red blood cells, white blood cells, and platelets are normal.

Blood Chemistries. This set of blood tests measures proteins and other dissolved materials. If a high level of the waste product uric acid is detected through this test, for example, it may indicate that gout is present.

Erythrocyte Sedimentation Rate. The more inflammation you experience, the more your body produces certain blood proteins that cause your red blood cells to clump together. These heavier clumps fall to the bottom of a vial of blood faster than normal red blood cells—a rate known as the "sed rate" or "ESR." The higher your sed rate, the more likely it is that you suffer from an inflammatory arthritis.

Rheumatoid Factor. This test is designed to detect the presence of an antibody known as rheumatoid factor, which has been found in about 80 percent of people with rheumatoid arthritis.

Synovial Fluid. Analysis of the fluid that fills the joint can provide a great deal of valuable information. Synovial fluid from a healthy joint is usually clear. When a doctor examines synovial fluid, he or she is looking for blood, bacteria, the number and kinds of white blood cells, and other material that would indicate that something is going wrong within the joint.

X-RAYS

X-rays are often a key tool in diagnosing arthritis because they allow the doctor to examine the swelling of soft tissue or fluid accumulation within the joint, as well as bone loss or changes in the surfaces of a joint. X-rays are especially helpful in helping the physician to distinguish between the two major types of arthritis: A joint beset by osteoarthritis is likely to have an irregular narrowing of its inner space, as well as a thickening of the bone and formation of cysts under the cartilage. Rheumatoid arthritis, on the other hand, causes a uniform narrowing of joint space, loss of bone density around the joint, bone destruction, and a swelling of the tissues.

ARTHROSCOPY

An arthroscope is a narrow fiberoptic instrument that is inserted into the body through a small incision. Severe swelling of the knees or shoulders may indicate the need for using the arthroscope, which allows the physician to see inside the joint in order to determine if damage has been done to the bone or cartilage. Although doctors do not commonly use arthroscopy as a diagnostic tool for arthritis, surgeons can use this instrument to perform surgery on the joints and to remove damaged cartilage or fluid from inside the joints.

Once your physician has determined the type of arthritis you have, he will attempt to devise a treatment plan designed to limit the pain and/or inflammation, preserve function of the joint, and prevent deformities. Unfortunately, mainstream medicine offers few options to the majority of people with arthritis, particularly over the long term.

Treating Arthritis

Generally speaking, mainstream medicine offers two alternatives to those with arthritis: long-term drug treatment or joint replacement and other surgery. Let's take a look each type of therapy to see what it might offer you:

DRUG TREATMENT

Two general classes of drugs are used in the treatment of arthritis: those designed to relieve pain and inflammation and those intended to limit or modify the progression of the disease.

Nonsteroidal Antiinflammatories (NSAIDs). This class of drugs, of which aspirin is the prototype, suppress (or reduce the degree of) inflammation in arthritic joints. NSAIDs usually provide pain relief quickly, sometimes within minutes, and can block inflammation if taken in high enough doses.

NSAID therapy, so long the standard arthritis remedy, is not without risk. The very action that makes NSAIDs so helpful in reducing pain is the same one that makes them so risky. This family of medications works by suppressing body chemicals called prostaglandins, hormonelike substances secreted by a variety of tissues that heighten pain and fuel inflammation. Unfortunately, prostaglandins also help protect the stomach lining, so when NSAIDs act to suppress their production, intestinal discomfort, bleeding, and formation of ulcers may occur, especially at the higher doses of pain relievers required by many people with arthritis. Each year, in fact, an estimated 20,000 to 50,000 people with arthritis develop treatment-related instestinal bleeding and more than 10,000 people die of related problems.

Apart from aspirin and other over-the-counter medications such as Advil, Nuprin, Aleve, and others, doctors may prescribe one or more of the following types of NSAIDs: salicylates (Ecotrin, Easprin, Trilisate, Salflex), ibuprofen (Motrin, Rufen), phenylbutazone (Butazolidin), indomethacin (Indocin), sulindac (Clinoril), naproxen (Naprosyn, Anaprox), piroxicam (Feldene), and etodolac (Lodine), among others. Although some of these drugs appear to have fewer side effects over the short term, when taken over time and at higher dosages, they may be equally disturbing to a patient's system. In addition, and more pertinently, NSAIDs may suppress cartilage growth, thereby slowing down a joint's healing process.

Disease-Modifying Drugs. Other types of drugs used to treat arthritis aim to suppress the overactive immune system. Unlike the NSAIDs, they do not offer immediate relief of pain and inflammation, but rather exert their effects slowly over time. (These drugs are generally not prescribed to people with osteoarthritis, a disease that generally does not involve inflammation.)

Currently, doctors prescribe several different disease-modifying drugs to people with arthritis: antimalarials (which help to suppress the immune system), gold compounds (used to reduce inflammation), a drug called penicillamine (which works to reduce inflammation by, some scientists believe, removing such heavy metals as copper, lead, and mercury from the blood), and sulfasalazine (a derivative of aspirin). For some people, one or more of these drugs may indeed help to stop the progression of their disease. A lot appears to depend on an individual's body chemistry and stage of disease. All of these drugs, however, have potentially damaging side effects, including skin rashes, kidney damage, anemia, and nausea, among others.

A large class of drugs known as corticosteroids are also used. Corticosteroids, including the widely prescribed prednisone, are a group of drugs similar in structure and function to natural hormones produced by the adrenal glands. These drugs, like the natural hormones, are used in the treatment of a wide range of inflammatory and allergic conditions, including asthma, autoimmune disorders, and arthritis. The drugs are also used to suppress the immune system so that the body does not reject a transplanted organ. Although corticosteroids are very effective in stopping pain and inflammation, they often have dangerous and unpleasant side effects. Because these drugs are so adept at suppressing immune function, many people taking them end up suffering from endless colds, flus, and other infections.

JOINT REPLACEMENT AND OTHER SURGERY

In recent decades, advances in surgical technology have made it possible to remove hips, knees, and wrists destroyed by arthritis and replace them with artificial joints. This type of surgery is usually attempted only when all other methods of relief have been attempted, although some doctors now suggest replacing wrists affected by rheumatoid arthritis early in the course of the disease, before deforming damage can occur in the soft tissue of the hands.

In addition to joint replacement, several other kinds of surgery help some people with arthritis. Synovectomy involves removing a diseased synovium, or joint lining. During an osteotomy, a surgeon cuts and then resets a joint into a better position. A resection involves removing of all or part of a damaged bone. And during arthrodesis, a joint is fused into a fixed position so that two bones don't rub together.

The surgical options open to you depend upon the type of arthritis you have, the joints involved, and your overall physical condition. With rare exceptions, joint surgery is not usually considered for people with lupus, gout or ankylosing spondylitis, and it should be considered a last resort for everyone else. Surgery itself is stressful and can be risky, often requires extensive recuperation and rehabilitation, and does not guarantee that the disease will not return or affect another joint.

As you can see, safe, effective treatment options for arthritis are few and far between. You may have come to an impasse in your own quest to find long-term relief and protection from further damage. Later in this book, you'll see how other schools of medicine, including those that developed in China and India, view the arthritic disease process and treatment. In the meantime, the next three chapters will show you the best foods to eat, the best ways to exercise and rest your joints, and the most effective methods of relaxing and relieving stress—habits that will work to help heal your joints while improving the general health of your body, mind, and spirit.

"All we know
is still infinitely
less than all
that still remains
unknown."

William Harvey

Choosing an Alternative

$\mathscr{A}$cupuncture. Herbal medicine. Homeopathy. Just a decade ago, such alternatives to mainstream diagnostic and therapeutic techniques formed a relatively small niche in the American health care market. Most of the American public—to say nothing of medical professionals themselves—appeared either unaware or uninterested in exploring these less "high-tech" methods of treating illness and disability.

In 1992, the National Institutes of Health, the federal government's largest supporter of biomedical research, announced the establishment of the Office of Alternative Medicine. Its goal was, and remains, to explore fresh approaches to such chronic degenerative diseases as cancer, AIDS, autoimmune disorders, and arthritis, for which standard medicine often offers no certain remedy. In part, the decision to open the office stemmed from the mounting evidence that increasing numbers of Americans seek alternative care every year—with or without the sanction of their mainstream doctors—for a whole host of minor and major illnesses and for a variety of reasons. Some try alternative medicine out of plain curiosity or because friends have recommended it. Most people go to a holistic practitioner, however, because they are searching for a new approach to healing their bodies and spirits. Alternative medicine is big business: American consumers spend upward of $15 billion every year on visits to acupuncturists, chiropractors, herbalists, and other holistic practitioners.

It is important to recognize, however, that to attain true health takes time and commitment. In addition, there are aspects of alternative health care that you may find unfamiliar and, at least at first, uncomfortable. Most forms of alternative therapy, for instance, require that you establish a more intimate physical relationship with your own body through exercise and massage. You may also have to become accustomed to being touched by a practitioner during examinations and treatment sessions far more extensively than usual, during both the diagnostic and treatment phases.

Furthermore, in order to gain the most benefit from natural medicine, you'll also need to learn to truly relax your body and mind. For many people, this experience involves exploring emotional and spiritual issues that they may have ignored or suppressed for many years. Although exciting, and ultimately healthful, such work will require special strength on your part, and support from both professionals and family members.

For the vast majority of people who choose to replace or supplement mainstream treatment with more natural methods, the benefits far outweigh the extra time and commitment. Later in this chapter, we'll outline some of the alternative approaches available to help you bring your body back into a state of more healthful balance, and in the process, help heal your arthritis. In the meantime, take the following quiz. It may help you to sort out some of the questions you have about alternative medicine and how it might, or might not, fit into your life. You may be surprised by what you learn.

Your Alternative Medicine Quick Quiz

The questions in this quiz focus on four different aspects of alternative medicine. The four questions in Part A focus on physical factors, Part B on nutrition, Part C on the emotional components of health, and Part D on practical matters. Answer yes or no to these questions, then check the answer guide to find out what you should look for—or look to avoid—when choosing an alternative therapy.

Part A
    1a. I enjoy being massaged or touched by a qualified practitioner. _____
    2a. I am willing to experience some discomfort during my treatment. _____
    3a. I have no fear of needles. _____
    4a. I enjoy physical exercise or am willing to make exercise a part of my life. _____

Part B
    1b. I am willing to change my diet. _____
    2b. I am willing to learn about nutrition. _____
    3b. I prepare most of my meals at home. _____
    4b. I accept that vitamins and minerals are helpful in treating disease. _____

Part C
    1c. I accept that emotions play a role in health and healing. _____
    2c. I am willing to explore my feelings. _____
    3c. I understand that restoring my body to health will take time and effort. _____
    4c. I now include meditation or relaxation routines as part of my daily life or would like to in the future. _____

Part D
    1d. I have easy access to one or more types of alternative medicine. _____
    2d. I have the time and desire to make and keep appointments for alternative treatments. _____
    3d. I have some discretionary income to pay for alternative treatments. _____
    4d. I can accept alternative therapies that have not been scientifically proven. _____

THE ANSWER GUIDE

Take a look at your answers. Were you able to answer most of them with a "yes"? Were there one or more categories in which you answered several questions with a "no"? As you'll see in the guide below, your answers to these questions will help you find the type or types of natural therapy that best suit your personality and needs.

A. The Physical. Many natural approaches to health care require people to establish a new relationship to their bodies and, in some cases, with their physicians and practitioners. If you dislike being touched by your doctor, then therapies that use physical manipulation as an integral part of their approach may not be for you. Likewise, if needles terrify you, then acupuncture may not be the method most helpful to you. Being tense while undergoing treatment works directly against the state of balance that is the goal of natural medicine.

However, because acupuncture, chiropractic, and massage are among the most effective alternative treatments for arthritis, it may behoove you to work through some of your fears and aversions with an understanding practitioner. He or she may also be able to help you use the philosophy behind the treatment without forcing you to undergo any form of treatment that makes you feel uncomfortable.

Finally, you will soon have to answer Question 4 with a resounding yes—with or without arthritis! Exercise must become a part of your life if you intend to stay active and mobile for the rest of your life. You must learn to keep your joints, tendons, and related structures as stretched and strong as possible with weight-bearing exercises and your heart strong through aerobics.

B. The Nutritional. Maintaining a healthy weight by eating the right kind of food in the right amounts is often a critical factor in the treatment of arthritis. Reducing fats, adding fiber, eliminating (or limiting) sugar and caffeine are just some of the dietary modifications you may need to make in order to bring your body into balance. In susceptible individuals, certain types of food may trigger or aggravate the process of inflammation, with its characteristic swelling, soreness, and stiffness. It will be up to you and the practitioner to work out the nutritional issues that apply to you.

As you'll see in Chapter 4, however, you should not feel over-whelmed by the thought of starting a "diet." We'll show you how to make changes in your eating habits slowly, over time, until they become natural and enjoyable.

C. The Emotional. Perhaps the most essential difference between mainstream and alternative medicine is the way in which the emotional side of life is considered. To understand and then to treat your particular case of arthritis, for instance, a holistic practitioner may ask you many questions about your sense of self-esteem, your family and professional relationships, and your ability to cope with the stresses in your life. Alternative practitioners consider these issues as important to making an accurate diagnosis and creating an effective treatment plan as the physical shape you are in or the condition of your joints and cartilage. Because emotional balance is an essential goal of natural medicine, it will help if you can learn to reduce the amount of stress in your life, as well as learn to better cope with and alleviate the stress that remains. To do so, however, you will need to invest time and energy in an area of your life you may well have neglected in the past. Chapter 6 will help you get started.

D. The Practical. In addition to the personal factors that may lead you toward a particular form of alternative health care, there are practical matters that you should consider as well. First and foremost is how much access you have to alternative resources. If you have to drive several hours to visit a homeopath or acupuncturist, treating a chronic condition like arthritis with these methods may not be possible. Time is another consideration. Many holistic therapies require more frequent visits to a practitioner than you may be used to; acupuncture and chiropractic are particularly time-consuming, as they usually necessitate continued, frequent appointments. Money is another obstacle for some people, since most forms of health insurance do not cover alternative medicine at this time.

Finally, another practical matter for you to consider is your own commitment to the process of natural healing. Many alternative therapies, despite having been practiced in other cultures for centuries, have not been proven according to Western medical standards. Even many Western drugs have not really been "proven" according to those ideal standards. Anyone who takes an aspirin for a headache can attest to that fact: sometimes it works, sometimes it doesn't. If you are someone who needs to understand the scientific basis for a therapy, some of these alternatives—homeopathy and Ayurvedic medicine, for instance—may seem too challenging for you at this time.

After considering these matters, and perhaps performing some additional research, you may narrow down your choices for alternative care to one or two options. No matter what type or types of natural therapy you choose, however, it is essential that you find qualified professionals to treat you. The following section offers a step-by-step guide to locating a reputable practitioner and establishing an effective supportive relationship with him.

Becoming a Wise Alternative Health Care Consumer

Successful treatment of arthritis, whether by alternative or mainstream means, requires a partnership between you and the people who treat you, one that is built on mutual trust and respect. You must feel confident in the practitioner's ability to treat your health problems, and she must have vital, accurate information about your medical status and lifestyle in order to provide you with that help.

Here are some guidelines to help you accomplish these goals:

Obtain an accurate diagnosis. Before you decide upon an alternative therapy or practitioner, you may require certain tests and procedures (see Chapter Two for more information). These tests are probably best performed either by your family practitioner or by a rheumatologist. Bring the results of these tests with you to your first appointment with an alternative practitioner.

Learn as much as possible about the alternative therapy or therapies that appeal to you. Knowledge is power, especially when it comes to health care. Read articles and books about the type of alternative care that appeals to you, talk to friends and acquaintances who use that method, and ask your mainstream physician for his or her opinion.

Check credentials carefully. Unlike those required for mainstream physicians, there are no national licensing requirements for most alternative medicine practitioners at this time. Instead, certification and licensing are done on a state by state basis. Ask your local department of health for the licensing requirements, certification, degrees, and diplomas suggested for a holistic practitioner. For more information about a specific treatment or a specific practitioner, you may call a national association in the specialty field you are considering. (See *Natural Resources*, page 168).

Interview your prospective practitioner. It is often a good idea to make a short "interview" appointment with a practitioner, even before you decide to be examined by her. During this visit, you should take note of the office itself: Is it clean? Do you feel comfortable there? What are the billing procedures and is the practitioner willing to set up a payment plan for you? Is the staff friendly and accommodating? Do patient boundaries and confidentiality seem to be respected?

When you meet with the practitioner, ask her how much experience she has had in treating arthritis. Find out how accessible she is in between appointments and in case of emergencies. Although it is doubtful that you'll feel completely at ease with the practitioner during this first short meeting, you should be able to tell whether or not there is potential for a close working relationship. Trust your instincts. If you feel uneasy for any reason, do not feel obligated to continue meeting with her.

Prepare for a long first appointment. Depending on the type of alternative therapy you've chosen to explore, your first appointment (after the prospective interview) may last from 45 to 90 minutes. You'll probably be asked detailed questions about your diet, your medical history, your exercise habits, and your feelings about the work you do and your personal life. Such information is crucial for the practitioner to have before she can develop a treatment plan for you.

At the same time, you should feel comfortable asking your own questions about your condition, about the procedures the practitioner intends to perform, and even about the questions she is asking of you. Your practitioner should answer these questions in an open and honest way. If you feel you are not being listened to or respected, you have reason to look for another person to treat you.

Get a clear idea of what the suggested course of treatment involves. Discuss what to expect from treatment *before* you agree to it. Ask the practitioner what to expect in terms of side effects or adverse reactions. Find out how many appointments and how much time it will take before you see symptoms alleviated. Ask how much the treatment will cost and if your insurance is likely to cover it. Although the course of treatment may change as therapy continues, a qualified practitioner should be able to give you a reasonable prognosis, timetable, and cost estimate.

Establish a relationship between your mainstream and alternative practitioners. Ask your mainstream doctor if he would be willing to collaborate with an alternative practitioner on your care— and ask the same thing of any natural therapist you choose. With a chronic, and fairly unpredictable, condition like arthritis, it is sensible to have access to the best of both worlds: the life-saving technology and pharmacology of Western medicine in cases of emergency and the more subtle, mind/body methods of healing implicit in alternative medicine. In Chapter Thirteen, you'll see how mainstream and alternative medicine can work together to bring you closer to true health—and to freedom from the pain your arthritis causes you.

Don't be afraid to experiment. What works for one person may not work for another, and that is especially true when it comes to health care. If the type of therapy you've chosen does not suit you for any reason, feel free to to explore another until you find one or more methods of health care and self-healing that work for you.

Now that you've received a primer of sorts on the basics of alternative medicine, it's time to explore the various techniques used to treat arthritis. In the next chapter, you'll find information about how what you eat may affect the health of your joints, tendons, and bones.

"A smiling
face is half
the meal."

Latvian proverb

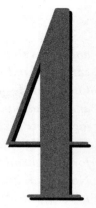

The Food Link

*J*eanne was overweight and knew that losing weight was the best way to address her continuing knee problems. Her struggle with the scale, however, had been lifelong. Meanwhile, her knees ached each morning and limited her mobility all day long. Her doctor told her that her last set of x-rays showed that the right knee was progressively on its way to an arthritis that eventually would require surgery to repair. The medications she now took, nonsteroidal anti-inflammatories, or NSAIDs, bothered her stomach. She decided to see a doctor who would treat her with more natural substances, a naturopath—a doctor who specializes in herbs and other natural treatments.

The naturopath examined her, took her medical history, then spoke to Jeanne about a diet that would allow her to take better control over her weight. Then, the doctor gave her a list of supplements *and herbs to take. Some called antioxidants, like vitamin C, beta-carotene, and vitamin E, are helpful in combatting joint damage. Other supplements were less familiar to her, including glucosamine and chondroitin sulfate, substances that the doctor said are essential ingredients in cartilage formation. Jeanne took these in capsule form, along with some vitamins and minerals. The doctor also gave Jeanne a form of vitamin B_3 called niacinamide, telling her how a physician in North Carolina, William Kaufmann, M.D., had shown niacinamide to be effective in osteoarthritis, especially of the knee.*

Within months, Jeanne felt the difference. There was less pain, less stiffness, and she had less difficulty getting up in the morning. Under her doctor's guidance, Jeanne began a walking and swimming program and began to shift her diet away from carbohydrates and starches—food that's good for many people but had been her particular downfall. As her weight dropped away, she became more motivated and energetic, even taking up an old hobby of hers, ballroom dancing.

Arthritis and food—the connection between the two has long been the subject of intense debate and research. Could what someone eats affect the health of their muscles, bones, and joints? Is there such a thing as an "antiarthritis diet"? Are there nutrients that are more helpful than others in suppressing the disease process and reducing pain? As this chapter explains, there does indeed appear to be a distinct link between food and inflammatory conditions, one that could mean a great deal to you in your struggle to find comfort and relief for your arthritis.

As you read this chapter, you'll probably be looking most closely at the specific suggestions we make about food and its relationship to arthritis. However, keep in mind that changing or supplementing your diet in order to improve the health of your joints will probably provide you with many other benefits, not the least of which will be a new sense of empowerment and self-esteem that comes with establishing any new positive habit. With every success, your spirit and energy—perhaps already a bit dampened and damaged by this chronic illness—will experience a renewal.

In this chapter, we'll explore three different ways that your diet may be affecting both your arthritis in particular and your general health. First, we'll look at the importance of maintaining a healthy weight in order to decrease stress and strain on the joints and muscles while providing you with a sensible, healthful eating plan. Then we'll outline the way allergies to certain foods may be triggering or exacerbating your disease process. Finally, we'll suggest a number of different vitamins and minerals that may help to relieve your pain, heal your joints, and prevent your arthritis from progressing.

Eating for Fitness and Health

Are you at a healthy weight, or are you like more than 30 percent of your fellow Americans: more than 10 percent over your ideal weight? If you are carrying extra pounds, they may be doing you more harm than simply bulking up your clothes or making you feel flabby. The extra weight could be contributing to the damage done to your joints by the arthritic process by forcing your joints to perform extra work to move this excess poundage. In fact, many researchers point to the increase in obesity as an important factor in the increase we've seen in cases of arthritis.

Why is obesity such a widespread problem in America today? Although most of us tend to blame our own lack of willpower, we can look to a number of outside influences that conspire to turn us into a nation of unhealthy eaters. Perhaps the most obvious and pervasive one is the television set. Not only does it compel us to spend too many hours sitting in a heap in front of it, but it constantly sells us apparently delicious, time-saving delectables—most of which are laden with fat and empty calories. The fact that our lives tend to be hectic and disjointed, leaving us with little time to plan our meals and enjoy them together with friends and family, also contributes to our increasingly poor eating habits and large waistlines.

At the same time, we read headlines every day about the dangers of food—sugar is bad, fat is worse, margarine is better than butter one day then a health risk the next. The mixed messages we receive tend to either confuse us to the point that we no longer even try to learn about nutrition or turn us into hypervigilant, slightly paranoid "food avoiders." In all this, we forget that food is good for us. It's meant to be enjoyed and savored at every meal.

Food is nourishment. The nutrients in the food you eat are the catalysts for millions of major and minor miracles—the beating of your heart, the birth of an idea, the appreciation of taste and smell—that take place within the chemistry lab that is your body. Food is also a source of pleasure. We do not eat merely to ingest the various vitamins, minerals, and other substances we need to survive. Instead, eating is a supremely sensual activity: We smell food's aromas, taste its flavors, admire its colors and textures, and feel its consistency inside our mouths. Depending on the circumstances, our sense of hearing is also stimulated by the conversation of our tablemates or the sounds of soothing dinner music.

As you consider your dietary habits, ask yourself these questions: Do you take the time to enjoy the sensual aspects of eating or do you think of food as simply fuel for the body? Or do you eat only those things that taste good without considering their nutritional value? Are there foods that you enjoy eating but which seem to exacerbate your arthritis symptoms or otherwise upset your system? Depending on how you answer these questions, you may discover that your approach to eating could use a little readjustment, especially if those habits have left you eating too much of the wrong kinds of food.

If you need to lose weight, or if you otherwise feel that you're not getting enough nutrition, take a look at the new Pyramid Plan devised by the United States Department of Agriculture. This plan organizes the food we eat into six different categories and shows us how much of each type of food we should, in general, eat every day. Please note, however, that your particular body chemistry may require more or less of certain foods in order to keep you healthy and arthritis-free.

> *Complex carbohydrates* (6 to 11 servings a day): Carbohydrates are substances that provide the body with energy, fiber, and the feeling of "fullness" we've come to expect from food.

Whole-grain bread, pasta, and rice are the primary forms of complex carbohydrates; most experts say they should compose the bulk of our daily caloric intake.

Protein (2 to 4 servings a day): Protein is the major component of our muscles and bones. In order for the health of our joints to be maintained, we need to consume some protein every day—about 55 grams, or the amount supplied in about 4 ounces of some lean meat, chicken, or fish. Among the most healthful sources of protein are cold-water fish such as mackerel, herring, and salmon, which contain certain substances called omega-3 fatty acids, which make anti-inflammatory substances in the body. Dr. Barry Sears, a researcher in metabolism, has recently pointed out that protein of any kind encourages the production of these anti-inflammatory substances in the body, while carbohydrates block their production. In his book, *Enter the Zone*, he suggests that a diet with 30 percent protein and 40 percent carbohydrate might be a better choice for a person coping with an inflammatory disease like arthritis. Research shows that several vegetable sources of protein, including some beans and legumes, provide other nutrients as well and may be better choices for those also attempting to lose weight.

Fruit (2 to 4 servings a day): The luscious sweetness of a peach, the exotic tang of a mango, the mellow tartness of fresh cherries. In addition to the pleasure we get from the flavor and texture of fruit, our bodies receive some essential nutrients from these foodstuffs, including antioxidants and flavonoids, two substances that work to keep body cells healthy and reduce inflammation.

Vegetables (3 to 5 servings, or more): "Eat your vegetables," our mothers told us, and like perhaps much of her other advice, this suggestion holds a great deal of merit. Vegetables provide the body with a wide variety of vitamins and minerals essential for its proper functioning, as well as fiber to help keep the digestive tract in good working order. We should all strive to eat more fresh vegetables every day.

Dairy products (2 to 3 servings): Milk, cheese, and yogurt are important to include in our daily diets because they contain calcium, magnesium, and vitamin D—all essential for the building and maintenance of our bones and muscles. For those of us who have difficulty digesting dairy products, there are other equally nutritious sources of these nutrients. Leafy green vegetables contain lots of calcium and magnesium, for instance, while fish and the rays of the sun provide us with vitamin D. Because fat inundates many dairy products, it's important to find some nondairy sources of these nutrients as well.

Fat and sugar (sparingly): From the foods listed above, we receive all the fat and sugar our bodies need to survive and thrive. However, as most of us can attest, fat and sugar, especially in combination, taste good. There are few among us who don't enjoy the sensual richness of chocolate or the mellow tartness of a lemon custard. As long as you limit the amount of these substances you eat on a regular basis, you should feel free—and guilt-free!—to enjoy an occasional treat (unless, of course, you have a medical condition like diabetes that involves specific dietary requirements). If you eat too much of these substances, however, it can have a definite impact on the arthritic process and the amount of pain and stiffness you feel for two reasons. First, you'll be more likely to gain weight—and thus place more stress and strain on your joints—if you overload on fat- and sugar-laden products. Second, as we'll see later in this chapter, sugar has a specific, and often quite negative, effect on the inflammatory process.

If you follow this rough outline—cutting way back on fat and sugar, eating more fresh fruit and vegetables, lean protein, and complex carbohydrates—it's likely you'll be able to maintain a healthy weight, even lose weight, even without counting calories. Nevertheless, knowing this simple fact may help you put weight loss into some perspective: *To lose weight, you must expend more calories than you consume.* Since 3,500 calories equal one pound of fat, you must either eat 3,500 fewer calories than your body needs to maintain its weight or burn 3,500 more calories through exercise to lose one pound. Indeed, another important fact to keep in mind is that exercise may very well be the key to staying healthy, fit, and able to eat the foods you love. Studies have shown that active thin people generally take in an average of 600 calories a day *more* than their overweight peers, proving the point that the amount of food you eat is not the only factor in losing weight. However, the key word is *active*: These people are working off more calories every day through exercise and the increase in metabolism that regular exercise induces. In Chapter 5, we discuss how to fit exercise into your life, even if arthritis besets your joints.

In the meantime, the simplest way to go about changing your diet in order to lose weight sensibly is to concentrate first on *adding* lots of good food. That's right. Losing weight does not always mean eating less and less food. You may be able to eat *as much* food as you ever have and still lose weight—if you eat the *right kind* of food. Our bodies use complex carbohydrates, for instance, much more efficiently than fat. A gram of fat provides more than twice the calories of a gram of carbohydrates (9 calories compared with 4). That's why one ounce of potato chips—processed in fat and totaling more than 160 calories—is more fattening than one ounce of baked potato, which contains about 30 calories and no fat at all.

In the end, then, the best way to diet is to concentrate on eating more vegetables, fruit, lean protein, and complex carbohydrates while cutting back on fat and sugar. If you eat relatively small portions of a wide variety of foods, and expect to lose just 1 to 2 pounds a week, you should be quickly on your way to improving your overall health and the health of your joints. Fad diets that promise rapid weight loss and focus on eating just a few select foods, on the other hand, are dangerous for many reasons. By concentrating solely on losing pounds and not on learning proper nutrition, you'll most likely fall back into the same kinds of bad eating habits that made you heavy in the first place. By adapting sensible portion control, you should be able to devise a healthy eating plan that will help you to lose or maintain weight without starving or depriving yourself of satisfying, filling foods. There are many such diet plans available, including those developed by Weight Watchers and the American Heart Association, if you need further guidance and support (see *Natural Resources,* page 168).

FINE-TUNING YOUR BODY CHEMISTRY

In addition to general dietary prescriptions for healthy eating, however, those with arthritis may need to look more closely at the amount of certain substances they ingest:

Antioxidants. Found in rich supply in fruits and vegetables, certain vitamins and minerals known as antioxidants appear to reduce the harmful effects of the inflammatory process by protecting muscle, tendon, and ligament cells from being damaged by chemicals called free radicals. Free radicals are unstable molecules created by normal chemical processes in the body (like the immune response to injury) or environmental influences like radiation and cigarette smoke. These unstable molecules, in an attempt to stabilize themselves, try to combine with other cells in the body. By doing so, they often damage the membranes and internal structures of healthy cells—including healthy muscle, tissue, and synovial cells—leaving them weak and unstable themselves.

In the body, the most damaging free radicals are derived from the chemical process by which oxygen is utilized inside the cells. Antioxidants, such as vitamins C and E, beta-carotene (which the body converts to vitamin A), and the mineral selenium, render these free radicals harmless. The more fresh fruits and vegetables containing these substances you consume, the better off your general health, and specifically the health of your joints, is likely to be. Later in the chapter, we'll discuss how you can boost your antioxidant levels by using vitamin and mineral supplements.

Flavonoids. The flavonoids are a group of plant pigments largely responsible for the colors of fruits and flowers. In addition, they serve to protect plants against environmental stress. In the human body, they modify the reaction to allergens and infectious agents. Flavonoids also have anti-inflammatory properties. Among the most important flavonoids for people with arthritis are those responsible for the colors of blueberries, blackberries, cherries, grapes, and other plants. Among their properties is the ability to increase vitamin C levels within cells, decrease the leakiness and breakage of small blood vessels, and protect against free radical damage. In addition, they appear to inhibit enzymes secreted by white blood cells that would otherwise destroy collagen structures during inflammation. Consuming the equivalent of a half pound of fresh cherries per day has been shown to be effective in lowering uric acid levels and preventing attacks of gout, as well as serving as a protection against the cell destruction involved in other types of arthritis.

Purines. Purines are natural substances found in certain foods, including organ meats, sardines, and anchovies. Research has shown that excess purine in the blood can raise uric acid levels. Uric acid, as you may remember from Chapter 2, has been directly linked to gout, a particularly painful form of arthritis. Excess uric acid may form crystals that settle in the joints, causing them to swell and, eventually, begin to erode. If you suffer from gout or another form of arthritis, most doctors would recommend that you limit the amount of purine-rich foods you eat.

Alcohol. To drink or not to drink? From its effects on atherosclerosis to cancer to arthritis, the impact of alcohol on disease remains the subject of a great deal of scrutiny among health professionals. Generally speaking, drinking a moderate amount of alcohol—about 2 to 4 ounces—every day appears to be good for most people (at least those who do not have an addictive problem related to alcohol). At least, drinking a small amount of alcohol appears to do no harm. As far as arthritis goes, however, there are a few exceptions. Alcohol may both increase uric acid production and reduce its excretion, which explains why alcohol consumption is often a precipitating factor in acute attacks of gout. Furthermore, heavy drinking—more than 4 to 8 ounces of alcohol a day—will deplete the body of a number of vitamins and minerals. However, if you currently enjoy an evening cocktail or a glass or two of wine with dinner and this habit appears not to cause a flare-up of your arthritis, you should feel free to continue to do so.

Sugar. When we eat simple sugars, such as refined table sugar or the sugar found in cookies and candy, the level of sugar in our blood (called glucose) rises rapidly. In response, the body releases a hormone, called insulin, which helps the cells absorb and use glucose as energy. If glucose and insulin levels rise and drop quickly, over and over again, muscle, tendon, and joint cells will become exhausted from these shifts. In addition, a chemical bonding occurs between muscle tissue, joint linings, and the sugar in the fluid that bathes them. This reaction, called glycosylation, goes on continually and irreversibly in direct proportion to the level of sugar in the blood. Hence, the more bonding that takes place, the more work your body tissues must perform. Therefore, the more sugar you consume, the more quickly your tissues will become damaged by this process. Finally, excess sugar in your diet and bloodstream may interfere with the proper functioning of your immune system. Should your immune system fail for this reason, infection may occur, further exhausting your body and leaving you open to aches and pain.

There is no need to deny yourself an occasional sugary indulgence if you have a sweet tooth. However, for many reasons, including those directly related to the pain, strain, and inflammation associated with arthritis, you should try to limit the amount of sugar you eat on a daily basis.

Now that you've read about some general guidelines related to diet and arthritis, it's time to look at the way food may be negatively affecting your individual body chemistry and disrupting the health of your joints and connective tissues.

Understanding the Food Allergy Connection

One man's nectar is another's poison—at least when it comes to the food we eat and the way it affects us. Some people are highly sensitive to certain foods, or substances in food, that may either trigger arthritis flare-ups or exacerbate the pain and inflammation involved. There is much evidence to show that an allergic hypersensitivity to certain foods or food-related substances can trigger arthritis in some individuals.

An allergy is an immune system reaction to a substance that most people find harmless. Your immune system is designed to defend your body against harmful organisms and substances, such as bacteria, viruses, and other invaders that cause infection. When the immune system recognizes a substance as being harmful, it mounts a response by producing white blood cells (called antibodies) and other chemicals that attack the offending substance.

If your immune system reacts to generally benign foreign substances, such as pollen, dust mites, or certain foods, you are said to be allergic to that material. When you come into contact with a food or environmental factor (such as pollen or molds) to which you are allergic, your immune system attacks it just as if it were a virus or bacterium. It releases a substance called histamine—a body chemical that can act as an irritating stimulant. When your cells release histamine into the lungs, it causes the lining of the airways to narrow, swell, and serete mucus. This leads to wheezing and coughing.

In some cases, histamine may be released into one or more joints, which causes an inflammatory response. This leads to arthritis-related swelling, tenderness, and stiffness that can become chronic and entrenched over time. Many scientists believe that a primary cause of rheumatoid arthritis may be food allergies, which trigger an autoimmune disturbance that results in the immune system attacking joint tissue.

Although you may be allergic or sensitive to any food, the most common culprits when it comes to back pain, especially back pain related to arthritis, are plants of the nightshade family—also called solanines—including tomatoes, potatoes, eggplant, and peppers. As discussed in Chapter 2, these foods tend to trigger the inflammatory response. Another plant of the nightshade family is tobacco. Not only might tobacco cause an allergic reaction, but nicotine reduces blood flow to the muscles and joints, further complicating matters for people with arthritis. Other common food allergies implicated in rheumatoid arthritis symptoms involve yeast and fermented products, wheat, and sugar.

If you are concerned that your symptoms are affected by food or other substances that you consume, talk to your doctor. She may suggest that you keep track of your diet and symptoms, writing down the foods you eat, when you eat them, and the symptoms that arise over the course of a day. After a few weeks, a pattern may appear. If a certain food appears to trigger an arthritis flare-up, it would, of course, make sense for you to avoid that food in the future.

In the end, the rule of thumb should be: "If it makes you feel bad, don't eat it!" Instead, eat the foods that contribute to your general health and sense of well-being, and avoid those that appear to intensify your symptoms or otherwise upset your system.

And if you smoke, stop as soon as you can. Talk to your health practitioner about natural herbs like chlorophyll and the amino acid L-glutamine, which may help you in your effort to beat the habit. Acupuncture, hypnosis, and biofeedback have all been used successfully in "stop-smoking" programs, but the first step is to sit down and really convince yourself that you want to stop. If you are trying to quit just because someone tells you it's bad for you, you probably won't be successful.

The ABCs of Nutritional Supplements

Although in the best of all possible worlds we would receive all the nutrients we need from the food we eat, many researchers believe that supplementing our diets with certain vitamins and minerals is an important component in any successful treatment of arthritis. The following nutrients are those most often mentioned in this connection.

Boron. Boron, a mineral deficient in most of our diets, may help prevent bone destruction such as occurs in osteopororsis. The usual supplemental dose is 3 to 6 milligrams a day.

Calcium and Magnesium. The mineral calcium is essential for bone, joint, muscle, and ligament health. Although it is only one factor in bone and joint maintenance, it is an important one. Your body does not produce any of its own calcium, so to meet your daily needs you must eat food rich in calcium or take calcium supplements. At the same time, however, you must also consume enough of the mineral magnesium, which allows bone tissue to absorb and use calcium. Without enough magnesium, any extra calcium in your blood ends up in soft tissues and joints, causing pain and swelling.

To bolster the supply you receive from fresh foods and to compensate for any deficiency, you should feel free to take up to 600 to 800 milligrams of magnesium a day. (Magnesium is found in high quantities in green leafy vegetables, nuts, and legumes.) As for calcium, you should consume at least 1,000 to 1,500 milligrams a day of this mineral or take a supplement to make up the difference.

Glucosamine Sulfate. Glucosamine is a naturally occurring substance found in high concentrations in joint structures. It appears that this chemical plays an integral part in stimulating the production of connective tissue and new cartilage growth essential to repair the damage done to these structures by arthritis. Research shows that as we age, we may lose the ability to manufacture enough glucosamine, resulting in damaged and weak cartilage that is then unable to hold water and act as a shock absorber.

When taken as a nutritional supplement, glucosamine sulfate appears to help the body to stimulate joint repair, thus reversing the arthritic process while reducing pain and inflammation. The standard dose for glucosamine sulfate is about 500 milligrams, three times a day. The body tolerates this supplement very well, much better than it does NSAIDs and other pain relievers, and thus may provide a welcome option for long-term osteoarthritis sufferers.

Omega-3 Fatty Acids. These fatty acids, derived mainly from cold-water fish such as mackerel and salmon, inhibit the inflammatory response. (In addition, omega-3 also helps to reduce cholesterol levels in the body.) If you wish to supplement your diet, you can take up to 10,000 millligrams per day. Make sure you purchase supplements that contain 150 to 1,000 milligrams of EPA, the active fatty acid in omega-3.

Pantothenic Acid. A member of the B-vitamin family, this micronutrient plays a key role in energy metabolism pathways in the body. It is also a component in the manufacture of cartilage. In addition, it is essential in the production of natural steroid hormones, necessary to keep our immune system up and running during times of physical and/or emotional stress. Egg yolks, kidney, liver, and fortified wheat flour are rich sources of pantothenic acid.

Selenium. This trace mineral is a component of an enzyme that is responsible for preventing the buildup of free radicals. By taking just 200 micrograms of this nutrient every day, you can help protect your muscles and bones from becoming damaged. Please note that selenium does not work alone: It requires sufficient amounts of vitamin E to function efficiently as an antioxidant. Selenium can be found in seafood and meats.

Vitamin B Complex. All of the B vitamins, including vitamins B_1, B_2, B_3, B_6, B_{12}, and folic acid, are considered important to the development and maintenance of bones and muscle, and thus essential to the health of one's joints. In addition, vitamins B_1, B_3, and B_6 are particularly helpful in reducing anxiety, which can help alleviate the cycle of pain that many people with arthritis must endure. Vitamin B_6 has also been shown to help reduce the pain of carpal tunnel syndrome, an impingement on the median nerve of the wrist and strain of the tendons of the hand and shoulder. Hence, it is quite possible that vitamin B_6 would also help to alleviate pain caused by similar functional problems in other joints afflicted by arthritis. A form of vitamin B_3, known as niacinamide, seems to have a positive effect on arthritis, especially of the knees. The usual dosage is 250 milligrams taken every few hours. Since niaicinamide may affect the liver, you should be under a doctor's care while taking B_3 supplements.

Foods rich in B vitamins include fish, nuts, grains, eggs, and lean meats. If you and your practitioner feel you aren't getting enough B vitamins in your diet, you may want to take 25 to 100 milligrams of vitamin B complex (available in both a one-dose time-release form and several smaller doses throughout the day). In addition, if your doctor suspects tendon involvement in your particular case of arthritis, you may want to add a dose of vitamin B_6, up to 10 to 50 milligrams per day.

Vitamins C, E, and Other Antioxidants. As discussed above, antioxidants help prevent the breakdown of body cells, including those of the muscles and joints. The stiffness you may feel when you try to move your joints during exercise, and the soreness you experience after strenuous activity, may be due in part to tissue-damaging oxygen molecules generated during exercise. These oxygen molecules attack the fats in muscle cell membranes, weakening the cells and leaving them open to further injury.

By increasing the amount of antioxidants you eat in fresh fruit and vegetables, as well as by taking vitamin supplements, you can thus help prevent your muscles, tendons, and joints from becoming damaged, inflamed, and sore. Recommended dosages of vitamin C supplements range from 250 to 3,000 milligrams per day. Please note, however, vitamin C can be quite acidic; the more you take, the more risk you have for developing stomach irritation, as well as diarrhea. Fortunately, it's possible to take forms of vitamin C, called ascorbates, which minimize this risk. Keep in mind that aspirin and other pain relievers tend to deplete the body of vitamin C, which is another reason you might want to supplement your daily intake of this vitamin. Recommended dosages of vitamin E supplements range from 200 to 800 international units per day.

Zinc. Studies in laboratory animals as well as in humans have shown that deficiencies in this trace mineral depress the immune system, leaving the body more vulnerable to infections—infections that could trigger the onset of arthritis flare-ups. Several studies show that the addition of about 200 milligrams of the supplement zinc sulfate improves mobility and decreases swelling in rheumatoid people with arthritis. Meat, liver, eggs, and seafood are the best dietary sources of zinc.

Now that you've read about how to improve your diet by avoiding foods that may be harmful to your health and eating foods that bolster your own internal health-promoting faculties, it's time to address another important issue: The amount and type of exercise you perform each day and the amount and quality of rest you provide your muscles, joints, and spirit.

"The harder you work, the luckier you feel."

Gary Player

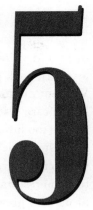

Exercise and Rest

$\mathcal{B}$y its very definition, arthritis is a disease that limits activity and laces movement with pain. It's no wonder, then, that those who suffer from its effects tend to neglect one of the most important health habits known to man or woman: exercise. The truth is, most Americans—even those without injury or disease—fail to provide their bodies with the physical exertion required to keep their bones strong, their muscles limber, their hearts and lungs healthy, and their joints supple. In fact, the results of a 1994 study performed by the National Center for Health Statistics showed that fewer than 50 percent of Americans perform any kind of exercise on a regular basis. Furthermore, the same study revealed that nearly one third of Americans remain obese—more than 20 percent above a healthy weight.

Overweight and underexercised, the human body leaves itself

open and vulnerable to a myriad of chronic conditions, including arthritis, back pain, heart disease, and diabetes, to name just a few. Without question, a large part of the current crisis in the American health care system derives from the mainstream medical community paying too little attention to the importance of fitness. Indeed, only in the past decade or so has the average general practitioner or, certainly, the average cardiologist or other specialist, emphasized the preventative and restorative power of exercise to his or her patients. For those of us who grew up before the message about exercise began to be enunciated as clearly and strongly as it has in the past few years, looking at the relationship between activity, health, and disease is a new experience. Hence, building exercise into our lives may seem like a tedious and difficult challenge.

At the same time, you may have noticed that the title of this chapter is "Exercise and *Rest.*" While it's true that exercise is extraordinarily important—so much so that information about exercise and arthritis makes up the overwhelming bulk of this chapter—resting your muscles, bones, and spirits is equally important to your health. The trick is, you cannot have one without the other. "Resting" an unstimulated mind or an underworked body leads not to renewal but to lethargy and weakness. You'll discover that rest, experienced at the right time and in the right ways, may feel far more invigorating and energizing than you imagine. In the meantime, however, we must examine the flip side of rest: activity.

Exercise and Your Health

Before we admonish ourselves for being lazy and unmotivated—as most of us do when we look at our general approach to activity and exercise—it is important that we recognize the powerful forces aligned against us on the road to health and fitness. First, the "miracles of modern medicine" have seduced many of us into believing that medication, surgery, and technology could protect us against the ravages of time and the environment. Furthermore, and perhaps most important, we live in a world driven by very mixed media messages about weight, body image, and lifestyle. We see rail-thin models advertising fat-laden potato chips and athletes peddling beer. Advertising prods us to buy time- and energy-saving devices like power-driven lawnmowers, snow shovels, and dishwashers. The television beckons to us constantly, urging us to relinquish the physical in favor of the passive. Too many of us give in to these temptations and spend from six to eight hours a day—every day—in front of the tube, while our automated appliances do our work for us. Thus our muscles grow weaker, our hearts give out sooner, our physical lives become more proscribed and limited.

Breaking out of this cycle of inactivity and chronic disease takes time, energy, and commitment. It also requires us to peel back the layers of misinformation, apathy, and frustration about health and fitness that may have built up over the years. Eating a proper diet *will* make you feel better and can be every bit as tasty and enticing as the foods you see advertised. Reading a book or learning a new language is *more* relaxing than passively watching television hour after hour.

And as for exercise, it is a positive life-enhancing habit that promotes physical and emotional well-being. It need not be a tedious grind or a painful ordeal. Properly performed on a regular basis, exercise allows you to connect with your physical body in an intimate way. You'll be able to feel your muscles grow stronger, your heart beat harder, and your nervous system throw off the built-up tension and stress of the day. Exercise will restore balance—balance within your body and balance between you and the physical world. With every hour we spend in the artificial environment promoted by television, fax machines, stuffy offices, and noisy factories, the further we get from nature and the true role we are meant to play within it.

What makes exercise so important? Let's take a look at the many different ways it affects our bodies and souls:

Exercise increases the efficiency of your heart and blood vessels. A primary function of your cardiovascular system involves transporting oxygen—an element essential to life—to every cell in your body. With regular aerobic exercise (exercise that requires oxygen for energy), your heart and vessels are able to pump more blood and thus deliver more oxygen and other nutrients to all the muscles and joints of your body. At the same time, the vessels known as veins, equally stimulated by exercise, carry away waste products, including excess calcium, uric acid, and other substances that might otherwise collect within your joints. Finally, exercise helps keep your blood pressure and blood cholesterol at normal levels, thus reducing your risk of heart disease and high blood pressure. Although not directly connected to arthritis, per se, these two chronic conditions remain the nation's number one health problem.

Exercise stretches joints and strengthens muscles. Of primary importance to those of us interested in preventing or alleviating arthritis is the development of supple, flexible joints and strong, lithe muscles. And, so far at least, the only way to do so is by using them every day and, on a regular basis, pushing them to their limits and a little beyond. Later in this chapter, we'll give you some tips on exercising safely and comfortably, even if arthritis has inflamed your joints and made them tender and difficult to move.

Exercise maintains your body's proper metabolism. More and more Americans suffer from obesity, which at least in part explains why arthritis is so prevalent. Every pound of extra weight places that much more stress on the joints, making them work that much harder, and promoting the kind of wear-and-tear degeneration associated with osteoarthritis, the most common form of the disease in the United States today.

With regular exercise, however, maintaining a healthy weight almost comes naturally, especially if paired with a sensible low-fat, high-fiber diet like the one described in Chapter 4. Through aerobic exercise, your body learns to burn stored fat more efficiently in order to meet its increased energy needs. Muscle tissue is more metabolically active than fat: Your body must burn more calories to feed and nourish muscle tissue than it would to maintain fat. Therefore, the more muscle you have, the more calories you'll burn every day.

Exercise allows the body and mind to relax. Stress plays a significant role in triggering arthritis flare-ups and perpetuating the cycle of pain once a flare-up begins. With tension comes tightness in the muscles and joints of the body and, if they fail to relax, they lose their suppleness. Over time, they may become permanently restricted and actually lose their ability to release and move naturally. Only by working your muscles and keeping your joints moving will the stress of the day (or the year!) ever be released.

Another mind/body benefit of exercise concerns certain body chemicals known as endorphins. Known to dull pain and invoke feelings of mild euphoria, endorphins are released whenever the body feels pain, including during vigorous exercise when the muscles begin to tire and "burn." Produced in the spinal cord and the brain, endorphins serve as a perfect example of the body's power to return itself to a state of balance. Indeed, endorphins may be one reason that exercise appears to reduce anxiety and stress in those who perform it on a regular basis.

For all of these reasons, you should begin to make exercise a part of your daily life. In this chapter, we briefly cover the three categories of exercise necessary to achieve overall fitness as well as help your joints to remain healthy and strong: stretching (range-of-motion), strengthening, and aerobics.

Devising an Exercise Plan

Now that you've read about the many benefits of exercise, you are (we hope) ready to make physical activity a regular part of your life. Before you jump in with both feet, however, it is essential that you speak first with your doctor or health practitioner, especially if you've been inactive in the past. Arthritis is a serious disease, one that has serious consequences for your muscles and joints. Depending on the state of your general health as well as the condition of joints, your physician may recommend that you first visit a physical therapist for an evaluation and advice. A physical therapist is a health professional with experience in working with people injured, ill, or otherwise physically restricted. He can take a look at the exercises we recommend in this book, offer you additional ones more suited to your needs, and help you perform all of them safely and in proper form. As careful as we might be to choose and describe appropriate exercises, nothing beats having someone watch the unique way your muscles work while you exercise, steer you to the exercises that will provide you with the most benefit, then make sure you're performing them efficiently.

STRETCHING

Many people neglect flexibility, even those who consider themselves to be in top physical condition. Part of the reason may lie in the noncompetitive nature of stretching: Unlike aerobics and weight training, there are no times or weight limits to beat. Instead, stretching the muscles and the joints they support, slowly and steadily to their limit and slightly beyond, requires an intensely personal effort, one that will bring you closer to truly understanding the unique structure of your own body. Stretching increases the range of motion of a joint, enriches the blood supply to the muscles, and brings important nutrients to the cells within and outside the joints.

If you have arthritis, range-of-motion or stretching exercises aim to move each of your joints as far as possible in all directions. They help keep your joints fully mobile and prevent stiffness, while decreasing the risk of the disease causing permanent deformities. Such exercises are especially important for those people with rheumatoid arthritis who tend not to want to move their inflamed joints. Lack of movement leaves the joints vulnerable to atrophy and even more pain.

Before we describe a few range-of-motion exercises, we want to stress the importance of performing a brief warm-up consisting of a few minutes of gentle jogging in place, riding on a stationary bicycle, or walking. Warming up in this way increases blood flow to the muscles and gets your heart started beating a little harder.

Once you've done your warm-up, you're ready to start taking your muscles and joints through a series of gentle stretches. When you stretch, you should never jerk or bounce. Instead, the movements should be slow and fluid. Try to hold each position for at least ten seconds, allowing the muscles and connective tissues to feel the full extent of the stretch. Do as many repetitions as you can manage—from 1 to 5 at the start to about 20—on each side.

Shoulder Stretch #1

1. Lie on your back, arms at your sides, and palms facing up.
2. Slide your right arm along the floor in an arc until you've raised it above your head.
3. Slowly bring it back down to your side.
4. Repeat with the left arm.

Shoulder Stretch #2

1. Lie on your back, arms at your sides, and palms facing your body.
2. Keeping your elbow straight but not locked, lift your right arm toward the ceiling until it is perpendicular to the floor. Hold for 10 seconds.
3. Slowly drop the arm down, again keeping your elbow straight, until it is lying on the floor again.
4. Repeat with your left arm.

Elbow Stretch

1. Lie flat on your back, placing your arms at your sides.
2. Keeping your upper right arm against the floor, bring your right hand as close to your shoulder as possible.
3. Hold this position for 10 seconds, then slowly lower it until the right elbow is completely straight.
4. Repeat on the left side.

Back Stretch #1

1. Lie on your back with your knees bent and your feet flat on the floor.
2. Tighten stomach and press your back against the floor. Try to feel every vertebrae making contact with the floor. Hold for 10 seconds, then relax.
3. Repeat.

Back Stretch #2

1. Lie on your back, with your knees bent and your lower back pressing into the floor.
2. Slowly lift both knees at the same time and bring them toward your chest.
3. Gently wrap your arms around your knees, pulling them in even closer.
4. Hold for 10 seconds, then release.

Hip Stretch #1

1. Lie on your back with your knees bent.
2. Lift your right leg, bending at the hip, raising your right knee toward your chest. Hold this stretch for 10 seconds, then slowly lower the right leg.
3. Repeat with the left leg.

Hip Stretch #2

1. Lie on your back with your knees bent and your feet flat on the floor.
2. Tighten your buttock muscles and lift your bottom and lower back up about 2 to 3 inches off the floor. Be careful not to push too hard with your shoulder or arm muscles.
3. Hold for 10 seconds, then slowly release.

Knee Stretch #1

1. Lie on your back with your legs straight. Try to straighten your right knee as flat as it can go by lifting your ankle and tightening the muscles around your knee.
2. Hold for 10 seconds, then slowly lower.
3. Repeat with your left knee.

Knee Stretch # 2

1. Lie flat on your stomach with your legs flat on the floor and your hands flat on the floor under your shoulders and elbows perpendicular to your chest.

2. Bend your right knee, aiming your right ankle toward your right buttock. When you've reached the extent of your stretch, hold for 10 seconds, then slowly lower the leg.
3. Repeat with left leg.

Ankle Stretch

1. Lie on your back with your legs straight.
2. Bend your right ankle, flexing your foot until your toes are pointing upward and your heel is pressing toward the wall in front of you. Hold for 10 seconds.
3. Release the flex, then point your toes as tightly forward as possible. Hold for 10 seconds.
4. Repeat with left leg.

Arch Stretch

1. Sit or stand with your right foot resting on a towel.
2. Attempt to pick up the towel by curling your toes and gathering the material under the arch of your foot. Clutch it as tightly as possible, then rest.
3. Repeat with your left foot.

Hand Stretch #1

1. Make a fist with your right hand, making sure to tuck your fingers into your palm.
2. Hold for 10 seconds.
3. Repeat with left hand.

Hand Stretch #2

1. Place your right hand and forearm flat on a table with your palm down.
2. Spread all five fingers as far apart as they'll go. Hold for 10 seconds.
3. Pull them together.
4. Repeat with left hand.

Wrist Stretch

1. Place your forearm flat on a table and dangle your wrist and hand over the edge.
2. Flex your wrist up as far as possible. Hold for 10 seconds.
3. Gently release.
4. Bend your wrist the other way, pointing your fingers toward the floor. Hold for 10 seconds, then release.
5. Repeat with your left wrist.

Depending on your current strength and desire for increased mobility, you may want to add the following stretches to your routine as well. Again, it's important for you to check with your doctor to make sure that working your body so thoroughly will not risk damage to your joints and muscles.

Shoulders/Upper Back Stretch

1. Raise your right arm and reach down your back as far as you can.
2. At the same time, reach your left arm behind your back and try to reach the fingers of your right hand. Hold the stretch for 10 seconds.
3. Repeat with your arms reversed.

Calf Stretch

1. Stand facing a wall, about an arm's length away. Lean forward on the balls of your feet, heels lifted, and bounce—very gently and only after you've warmed up!—20 times.
2. Place your palms on the wall, leaning forward slightly, but this time, keeping your heels firmly planted on the floor. Hold this stretch for 10 seconds.

Hamstrings

1. Stand up straight. Place your right foot about 12 inches in front of your left foot.
2. Try to raise your right toes in the air.

3. Keeping both knees slightly bent, lean your torso forward as if to take a bow.
4. Feel the stretch in the back and front of your thigh for about 10 seconds.
5. Reverse the position, leading with your left foot.

STRENGTHENING EXERCISES

If you have arthritis, strengthening the muscles that support the joints involved in the disease process is essential. In addition, overall muscle strength and endurance are critical to your general health and fitness. Indeed, every muscle in your body plays a vital role in keeping you standing tall, moving smoothly, and maintaining your balance.

We achieve muscle strength and endurance by applying resistance to normal body motion. The resistance, or load, causes muscles to contract at an increased tension. We add resistance in two ways: through the weight of our own bodies in a series of exercises called calisthenics (sit-ups, push-ups, and so forth) and by using hand-held or adjustable weights. Because the techniques of calisthenics and weight training are very precise and, if not performed correctly, can lead to injury, we suggest that you visit a local gym or YMCA to receive firsthand instruction before you begin a program on your own.

A weight-training routine should involve about 30 minutes of slow but constant stress on different muscles of the body using your own body weight (calisthenics), free weights, or strength-training equipment (such as Nautilus). An exercise specialist familiar with your limitations and goals should help you formulate a complete strength-training routine. Generally speaking, however, you should perform about a dozen exercises, six for the upper body and six for the lower.

Please note: Anaerobic exercises, including calisthenics and weight training, are usually not recommended for people with high blood pressure or other types of cardiovascular disease. Such exercises may cause temporary but marked rises in blood pressure. If you suffer from high blood pressure or heart disease, or if you are over the age of 40 and are new to weight training, talk to your physician and/or alternative practitioner before beginning a routine.

ENDURANCE EXERCISE

Endurance exercises, also known as aerobic exercises, are those activities that promote cardiovascular fitness by enhancing your body's ability to deliver large amounts of oxygen to working muscles. Aerobic exercises generally involve working large muscle groups (such as leg muscles) for a sustained length of time, usually more than 20 minutes, at a steady, moderate pace. In addition to furthering cardiovascular health, aerobic exercise increases your body's ability to burn fat more efficiently and deliver more nutrient-rich oxygen and blood to joint tissue and muscles.

It should be noted that not all people with arthritis are able to perform endurance exercises. Those who have had rheumatoid arthritis for many years and thus already suffer many functional limitations, for instance, may not be able to participate in this type of activity. Generally speaking, however, most people with early- to middle-stage arthritis of any type will benefit from adding endurance exercise to their lives.

At the same time, you should choose an endurance exercise carefully in order to avoid further injuring already affected joints. For that reason, the vigorous jumping and pounding involved in city jogging or high-impact aerobics should be avoided by those with arthritis, especially arthritis that affects the feet, ankles, and/or knees.

There are literally dozens of safe and enjoyable activities that can provide aerobic benefits if performed over a sustained period of time— at least 15 to 30 minutes—including walking, cycling, and swimming. Some activities, however, tend to involve a bit more risk to the joints than others, and thus should be undertaken with extreme care. If you enjoy a sport or exercise that you find to be painful or if you are fearful that pain might occur if you attempt it, talk to a trained physical therapist or fitness trainer. She may be able to help you modify the activity or work with you until you feel more comfortable.

Remember, a prime benefit of exercise is the sense of release and relaxation it offers. You should enjoy this time of your day, not be held prisoner by either the activity itself or any anxiety you feel about performing it. To help you on your way to a creating a safe and enjoyable exercise routine, we provide a list of the most common aerobic activities along with a description of how they might affect a person with arthritis:

LOW-RISK ACTIVITIES

Walking. Perhaps the best overall exercise for every adult, with or without arthritis, walking puts less strain on the joints of the hips, knees, back, and feet than jogging, running, or cycling.

Swimming. Because water supports the joints, swimming tends to relieve pressure while putting your muscles through a full range of motion.

Bicycling. Stationary or outdoor cycling is an excellent aerobic exercise that can usually be performed without adding too much stress to your joints. The one exception involves those who have severe knee problems who may find this exercise too difficult and stressful on these joints. If you decide to try cycling, make sure to adjust the handlebars and seat so that you don't have to hunch over when you pedal or overextend your limbs (locking your elbows, knees, and/or wrists, for example).

HIGHER-RISK ACTIVITIES

Jogging/Running. These activities place a great deal of stress on the joints of the ankles, knees, and hips. Unless running is your passion and you've talked the matter over with your doctor and a fitness trainer, you might do best to choose another aerobic activity.

Tennis and Other Racquet Sports. Tennis, racquetball, and squash require a great deal of twisting, turning, and pivoting of the hips and legs, as well as plenty of sudden starts and stops. The grip required to hold the racquet and the stress that hitting the ball places on your elbows and shoulders are other potential challenges of taking up a racquet sport. On the other hand, these sports are fun, can provide aerobic benefits if performed at a sufficient level of play, and certainly work important muscles like the shoulders, chest, hip flexors, and quadriceps. If one of these activities interests you, ask advice from your doctor and/or a fitness trainer.

Football, Basketball, Baseball. Apart from the bending, lifting, and stop-and-start aspects of play that may affect any arthritis in your spinal column or hips, these sports often involve sliding, falling, jumping, and contact with other players. If your joints are already weak and/or inflamed, it might be best to avoid these activities unless you have your doctor's permission.

General Exercise Guidelines

In the best of all possible worlds, every one of us would get out of bed bright and early, take a few deep breaths, run in place for a few minutes, gently stretch our muscles, then take a brisk walk, a short jog, or a play a set of tennis. But for most of us, that scenario is not a reality. Instead, we must work exercise into our lives, slowly but surely making it part of our weekly, if not our daily routine.

To start, we suggest concentrating first on performing the stretching exercises outlined in this chapter—every day if possible. This way, you'll be sure to keep your joints as supple and flexible as possible, even if you can't yet add strength training or endurance exercises to your routine. Once you're able, try to exercise aerobically for at least 30 minutes at least three times a week, then add a half-hour of strength training on the days you aren't jogging or swimming.

Above all, don't get discouraged if you are not able to meet this schedule at first: Every time you move your body—even if it's for just 10 minutes a day—you're doing something positive for you health. On the other hand, to really experience a difference in the way you feel about your body and your health, you'll need to make exercise a regular part of your life.

Here are a few tips to get you started on the road to fitness:

Check with your doctor or practitioner. Your first step in starting any exercise program is to consult with your physician and/or alternative practitioner, especially if you're overweight, suffer from late-stage arthritis, or have any risk factors for cardiovascular disease.

Start slow. A study published in the *Journal of the American Medical Association* in November 1989 showed that moderate exercise—defined as 30 minutes a day of light activity such as walking and gardening—is almost as beneficial to one's health as higher levels of exercise, such as high-impact aerobics and jogging. Moreover, moderate exercise is far safer than high-intensity activities for those people whose joints have already been damaged by the arthritic process.

Choose activities you enjoy. Perhaps the most important element in the design of your exercise program is choosing activities you will enjoy over the long haul. Think of it this way: If you exercise three times a week for 30 minutes a session, you'll have jogged, danced, or walked for about 78 hours—the equivalent of two solid workweeks—by the end of the year.

Wear proper footwear. Although there is no need for you to spend lots of money on fancy walking shoes or aerobic sneakers, you should choose a shoe that has a rigid arch and some cushioning on the heel and ball of the foot. Such support will help keep your body properly aligned and thus less likely to place undue stress on your ankle, knee, or hip joints as you exercise.

Set realistic goals. If you've been sedentary for a number of months or years, deciding to train for next month's marathon by running ten miles every morning would be counterproductive and even dangerous, especially if you have arthritis. After failing to meet the unrealistic goal, maybe damaging your knees or hips trying to do so, you'd most likely become too frustrated and discouraged to exercise at all. Instead, set goals you know you can meet, or perhaps ones just out of reach. Achieving them will give you a sense of pride and self-confidence, emotions that are sure to motivate you further.

Vary your routine. Plan two or three different workout routines in addition to stretching every day. Bicycle one day, walk the next, try a new sport (once you've checked with your doctor) the next. This will cut back on the chances you'll get bored with your exercise program, a prime reason that many of us end up relinquishing our newfound habits.

Find support. For most of us, there comes a time when our

motivation sags and we lose interest in exercising on a regular basis. When this happens—preferably *before* this happens—enlist a friend or a loved one to join you in your fitness quest. Join a gym or a walking club—or start one on your own.

The Importance of Rest

So far, we've concentrated most on the essential role that exercise plays in maintaining general health and in helping joints plagued by arthritis stay as limber and strong as possible. Without question, you run a higher risk of sinking into illness and disability if you fail to keep active than if you give in to the quite natural inclination to pamper yourself with long periods of complete rest.

On the other hand, exercise specialists and rheumatologists alike long ago discarded the notion of "no pain, no gain." Indeed, pain is the body's way of signaling that something has gone awry, and to ignore that signal is to risk further injury to your joints. If you feel pain every time you flex your wrist or bend your knees, then playing a game of tennis is likely to be both exceedingly unpleasant and potentially quite dangerous. That's not to say, however, that you shouldn't feel challenged—aerobically and strengthwise—when you exercise. You should be taking larger, deeper breaths than usual at the height of your exercise session, and your muscles and joints should work to their capacity, which may leave them feeling fatigued.

However, should you experience sharp pain, shortness of breath, chest discomfort, or dizziness at any time during your session, stop exercising immediately and tell your doctor or fitness trainer about your symptoms. If you're just beginning to exercise after a long sedentary spell, feel free to take frequent breaks during the exercise period. Finally, if you feel fatigued for more than two hours after an exercise session or if you are unable to flex and stretch your muscles freely the next day, chances are that you've pushed yourself too hard too fast.

Take it a bit easier and build up to a challenging but not taxing level of endurance slowly over time.

Treat yourself—and your joints—to some true comfort and rest. If your joints feel hot and swollen, cool them off by holding an ice pack on them for 15 or 20 minutes, especially after strenuous exercise. If inflammation and swelling aren't involved, take a long, warm bath, then massage your muscles and joints to bring blood and precious nutrients to the rescue.

Finally, and most important, use the time spent both exercising and resting to truly relax your mind and spirit. As we'll discuss more thoroughly in the next chapter, stress, tension, and negativity can weigh your joints down as much as any excess poundage. Indeed, as you may yourself have experienced already, the inflammatory response itself is quite often triggered by anxiety, anger, or emotional upheaval of any kind. Chapter 6 introduces several methods of meditation and relaxation that may help you to release the stress you now hold inside.

"He who

laughs, lasts."

Anonymous

Releasing Pain
through Relaxation

*A*t first glance, it may surprise you to see a chapter about meditation in a book about a rather mundane, nitty-gritty disease like arthritis. Like most Americans, your parents and teachers probably taught you to believe that what happens in your brain (or spirit) has little to do with the rest of your body. Arthritis, after all, directly attacks the joints and connective tissues while meditation, on the other hand, involves only the brain and the breath.

Fortunately, a new understanding of the major role that emotions play in our physical lives has begun to emerge, even from the most hard-core modern medical centers. Indeed, we now know that the way we feel, on an emotional and spiritual level, affects everything from the ability of the gastrointestinal tract to digest food properly to the intensity and frequency of the inflammatory response within our muscles and joints. In this chapter, we'll show you ways to harness the wonderful healing power you hold within your own heart and mind. First, though, we want to give you a better understanding of what pain is, and how its vicious cycle might be working to undermine your emotional and physical health.

Mapping the Pathways of Pain

There are two basic types of pain: acute and chronic. Acute pain is a warning, a message from the body that something is wrong and needs attention. When you put your finger on a hot stove, for instance, the ensuing pain causes you to pull back, protecting yourself from becoming seriously burned. Acute pain eventually resolves itself when the danger has passed and the trigger has been released. Another example of acute pain might involve an elbow joint already severely damaged by osteoarthritis. Hitting a squash ball using a racquet held by that arm would cause great pain because the bones of the arm now rub together instead of being cushioned by healthy cartilage and lubricated by synovial fluid. The pain would cause you to stop playing squash, and thus you would avoid further injury to your elbow joint. That's why it's so important that we listen to our pain and heed its warning signal.

Chronic pain, on the other hand, continues for long periods of time and, apparently, serves no useful physiological function. With a long-lasting and variable condition like arthritis, you can literally become "stuck" within the pain, caught in a cycle of frustration, fear, and exhaustion. You hurt your elbow playing squash. The next day it still aches. You become afraid of straining it further, so afraid that you try not to move it at all. Whenever you do, it seems to hurt even more. Every movement becomes a struggle, a struggle that finally undermines your confidence and energy. Eventually, you become stuck within this cycle, unable to free yourself from the psychological damage that the initial pain and injury wrought.

This is not to say that chronic pain is any less real or serious than acute pain. In fact, chronic pain may point to deeper, more intractable physical and emotional problems, problems that require more, not less, attention and commitment on the part of the individual and his or her practitioner to treat. And, acute or chronic, pain is a very individual and personal matter. No two people experience pain or find relief from it in exactly the same way. Although a fracture of the wrist bone or a cavity in a molar appears to do the same amount of damage in any two individuals, the way pain is perceived by each of them may be completely different: One might be in agony while the other complains of only minor discomfort. This makes the treatment of pain a particular challenge.

Keep in mind that the word "perception" is an important one when it comes to a discussion of pain and our response to it. That's because the pathway from stimulation (injury) to response (ouch!) is not a straight one. When you burn your finger on a stove, for instance, the sensation of pain travels along a series of nerve fibers from your finger to the brain. And there are many ways that the pain message may be altered or even canceled along the route. Have you noticed that when you're in a hurry or preoccupied, stubbing your toe is only a minor interruption, while on other days, perhaps when you're more (or less) relaxed, the same minor injury feels excruciating? Such differences in our own perception of pain point to the complexity of the pain pathways.

Perhaps the most important way that the body protects itself against pain is by producing substances called endorphins. Endorphins are chemicals produced in the brain, spinal cord, and elsewhere in the body in response to the perception of pain. Once released, these chemicals are able to attach to certain receptors in the brain and other sites in the body, thereby dulling the perception of pain. In fact, opiates such as morphine and heroin have a chemical structure similar to that of endorphins, which accounts for their painkilling capacities.

The brain produces endorphins under a number of different conditions, including exercise, meditation, and the stimulation of acupuncture points. In addition, certain emotions and emotional responses appear to either trigger or hinder the release of endorphins. Some studies indicate that depression, a common side effect of chronic pain, for instance, decreases endorphin production, while laughter increases production.

Self-esteem is an extremely important, and often overlooked, aspect of health. Those who feel that they are destined to fail (and thus have no control over their lives) or are unworthy of the success they do achieve, tend to feel stress and pain more acutely than others with more confidence in themselves and their ability to alter their environments. Indeed, our emotional lives have a direct bearing on all aspects of our physical health, including the state of the muscles, tendons, and nerves.

Arthritis and Stress: The Connection

Once your brain perceives pain of any kind, several different hormones are produced that stimulate a number of physical and emotional reactions. When you are frightened by the pain or what caused it, for instance, your palms may begin to sweat, your heart rate and blood pressure to rise, and your muscles to contract. Known as the "fight-or-flight" response, this is an automatic reaction meant to keep you safe from any situation that you perceive of as dangerous. It prepares us to either stay and fight the "enemy," in this case whatever triggered the pain, or to flee. When this response is triggered over and over again by chronic pain, the end result may be more harmful than protective, however. It is, in fact, another form of stress that can weigh heavily on your mind and body.

One branch of the nervous system, called the autonomic nervous system, is particularly important in the fight-or-flight stress response. The autonomic nervous system regulates bodily functions like the heartbeat, intestinal movements, muscular contraction, and other activities of the internal organs. It is divided into two parts that work to balance these activities: The sympathetic nervous system speeds up heart rate, raises blood pressure, and tenses muscles during times of physical or emotional stress, while the parasympathetic nervous system works to slow these processes down when the body perceives that the stress has passed.

Indeed, the two parts of the autonomic system represent a perfect example of the balance we know of as health. (In Chinese medicine, the sympathetic nervous system is the "yang" and the parasympathetic system is the "yin" of the body and its responses.) Bringing your body into harmony during and after stressful periods by triggering your parasympathetic nervous system is as important to your health as is reacting immediately, through the sympathetic nervous system, to the perceived threats known as stressors.

Two of the most powerful stress-related hormones are called norepinephrine and epinephrine. These hormones stimulate the sympathetic nervous system to raise blood pressure and heart rate, to make you breathe in more oxygen, and to cause your muscles to tense up. If you remain under constant pain, the muscles that support your joints and the joint tissues themselves may become chronically and abnormally contracted and thus achy or subject to spasm.

At the same time, the more stress and pain you feel, the more likely it is that you will engage in high-risk behaviors, such as smoking and drinking, overeating, and exercising too little. Although you may feel that these habits help to relax you, they are, in fact, increasing the stress on your body by forcing you to cope with the ill effects of these substances and behaviors.

The good news, however, is that within our bodies we have powerful weapons that can fight against chronic pain and stress. In short, we are naturally able to both boost our production of the natural painkillers called endorphins and, often at the same time, reduce the amount of debilitating, pain-producing "fight-or-flight" responses.

Controlling Pain through Stress Reduction

Although you may be under the impression that what you need to alleviate your arthritis is ever more powerful drugs, it is unlikely that medication will ultimately solve your problem if you remain under high levels of emotional and physical stress. At the same time that you undergo other treatment for your pain, you may want to examine some of the stress-related factors that may well be causing, or at least contributing to, your condition.

Is job stress undermining your health? What about your relationships? Your lack of physical activity? Do you live in a hostile environment, either physically or emotionally? If you can answer yes to any of these questions, you might want to consider ways to change your life in order to eliminate or at least alleviate these problems. Is it possible to change your job? Could you spare the time and money to receive family therapy to improve the way you relate to those close to you? Can you make stretching and strengthening exercises such as those that were described in Chapter 5 a regular part of your life? Although making such fundamental changes may take a great deal of time and commitment on your part, the impact on your general state of fitness and health is likely to be enormous.

In the meantime, there are several other—perhaps more practical—methods of stress reduction available to help you to bring your body back into balance quickly and efficiently during times of stress. In essence, you can learn to counteract the "fight-or-flight response" by activating your parasympathetic nervous system—your yin to counteract the overactive yang sympathetic nervous system—to attain a more peaceful and relaxed internal harmony. Biofeedback, hypnotherapy, guided imagery, meditation, and progressive relaxation are just a few of the many techniques known to help release physical and emotional tension. You should try a few different methods, each one for a week or two, before deciding which ones work best for you.

BIOFEEDBACK

Biofeedback is a time-tested, scientific method for exploring and utilizing the mind-body connection. It is especially helpful for chronic pain sufferers, like the majority of people with arthritis, who can learn to use the power of their own mind to control and release their pain. The underlying premise behind biofeedback is that anyone can learn to modify his own vital functions—including heart rate, blood pressure, and muscle tension—by using his conscious mind. In other words, when properly trained, you can learn to relax your muscles and release the stress such tension can cause your joints whenever you feel tightness and constriction beginning to take hold.

Scientists first developed biofeedback after conducting studies that showed how animals could control bodily functions once thought to be completely automatic by being given a reward or a punishment. Physicians adapted those findings to design ways for humans to control unconscious functions through conscious thought. For thousands of people with arthritis and others with chronic pain, this technique has spelled the end to years of frustration and pain.

Although there are several biofeedback methods, they all have three things in common: one, they measure a physiological function such as muscle tension; two, they convert this measurement to an understandable form such as a computer-generated graph or chart, a blinking light, mercury levels in a thermometer; and three, they feed back this information to the patient.

As with all aspects of health care, it is important that you receive biofeedback therapy from a qualified practitioner. Generally speaking, that means someone with a firm grasp of both physiology and psychology who has been certified by the Biofeedback Certification Institute of America.

HYPNOTHERAPY

Hypnosis, or hypnotherapy, is a technique named for Hypnos, the Greek god of sleep. Since 1958, when the American Medical Association officially approved hypnotherapy as a tool for treating back pain, thousands of people have benefitted from its physically relaxing and emotionally releasing effects.

The goal of hypnotherapy is to bring your body and mind into a deeply relaxed state in order to make you more open to suggestion. Usually, a hypnotherapy session begins with the therapist asking you to close your eyes and think relaxing thoughts. With a soothing voice, the therapist guides you down a path of deeper and deeper relaxation by asking you to focus your attention on a word or an image. By doing so, the therapist hopes to quiet your conscious mind and to make the unconscious mind more accessible by blocking all outside thoughts and stimuli. Because the unconscious mind is less critical, suggestions have a better chance of taking effect than they would if you remained in a normal, alert state.

Once you are completely relaxed, the therapist may suggest that you experience your joint and muscle pain in a different, more pleasant way, or that you picture the pain flowing out of your body in a stream. The therapist may also plant posthypnotic sugges- tions—ideas about your pain and pain relief that take effect after you return to full waking consciousness. These suggestions are designed to help you release the pain whenever it occurs. In the end, the ultimate goal is to give you a greater sense of control over your own discomfort and frustration.

When choosing a hypnotherapist, you should ask your doctor for suggestions as well as check with national training and licensing insti- tutions, such as the American Institute of Hypnotherapy and the Inter- national Medical and Dental Hypnotherapy Association.

GUIDED IMAGERY

Another form of treatment for chronic pain, called guided imagery, uses the power of the human mind as its basic tool. The human imagi- nation—that part of our hearts and minds that can picture and sense images and feelings—is one of the most potent health resources we have available to us. By utilizing the power of the mind, we can help evoke a physical response in our bodies in order to relax our muscles, stimulate (or depress) our immune systems, and reduce pain. In fact, guided imagery is now being used to treat any number of conditions in addition to arthritis, including chronic back pain, high blood pressure, gastrointestinal disorders, allergies, and premenstrual syndrome.

In addition to helping you relax your body, guided imagery also helps to access your emotions. By visualizing your arthritis pain as a red and angry monster that you imagine banishing from your king- dom, for instance, you may learn to better understand how frustrated and sore the pain has made you feel, and how powerful and in control of your body you can be if given the chance to break the cycle.

Although it is possible to conduct your own guided imagery session, it is best when learning to have a trained professional, preferably someone who has experience with your particular type of arthritis, develop a program for you and guide you through the steps until they become familiar. Talk to your doctor about finding a qualified therapist for you.

MEDITATION

Like biofeedback, hypnotherapy, and guided imagery, meditation is a mental exercise that affects body processes. The purpose of meditation for relaxation is to gain control over your thoughts so that you can choose what to focus upon and thus to let the stress flow out of your body. Meditation for relaxation requires no special training, and can be done at any time of day and in any comfortable space. All it takes is about 15 minutes of uninterrupted quiet.

Meditation is effective both in reducing general stress and in helping to relax muscles and joints made tense by anxiety or worry. When you meditate, you quiet the sympathetic nervous system, thereby reducing the heart rate and state of muscle contraction. In addition to its physical benefits, meditation can help you psychologically by allowing you to focus on the cause of your stress and find ways to change the way you respond to the challenges you face. Researchers have found that meditation is related to an internal locus of control, greater self-actualization, more positive feelings after encountering a stressful situation, improvement in sleep behavior, and even an increased ability to quit smoking.

There are many good books on meditation available on the market that go into great detail about the proper sitting positions, what to expect, even what to chant, if you want to chant. And there are schools of meditation that train both doctors and lay people in the intricacies of the meditative process. But the basic elements of meditation are very simple, and can be mastered by anyone willing to set aside a few minutes a day. An easy meditation exercise follows:

Basic Meditation Exercise

This is a simple meditation exercise that can help you relax and focus your attention away from the things that cause stress in your life. Start by sitting a few minutes—perhaps just 5 to 10—until the practice becomes comfortable to you. (If you are interested in learning more about meditation, see *Natural Resources*, page 168.)

1. Make sure you are wearing comfortable, loose, nonbinding clothing. Sweatpants or shorts and a T-shirt are ideal.
2. Find a quiet place where you will not be disturbed. Try not to sit any place where you might be easily distracted, such as in front of a window.
3. Sit on the floor in a comfortable position. If you aren't comfortable sitting on the floor, sit in a straight-backed chair.
4. Allow your hands to rest on your legs.
5. Lower your gaze so that your eyes are almost, but not quite, closed.
6. Take a deep breath and let it out slowly.
7. The easiest way to begin meditation is to count your breaths. Inhale, count one. Exhale, count two. Inhale, count three. Exhale, count four. Do this to ten, and then start again with one.
8. Sit for about 5 minutes the first week or so (try timing yourself with a kitchen timer so that you don't have to keep track of the time). Gradually increase the time you meditate to 15 to 30 minutes a day.

PROGRESSIVE RELAXATION

Progressive relaxation is a technique used to induce nerve-muscle relaxation. It was developed by Edmund Jacobson, M.D., a physician who designed the technique for nervous hospital patients. It involves tensing one muscle group, then relaxing it, slowly moving from one muscle group to another. The purpose of first contracting the muscle is to teach people to recognize more readily what muscle tension feels like. The idea is to sense more readily when we are muscularly tense and then learn to relax the muscles. Progressive relaxation has psychological benefits as well. Studies show that self-esteem is raised, depression lessened, and sleep problems alleviated in people who practice this relaxation method over a period of several weeks.

Usually, a progressive relaxation session begins by tensing then releasing the muscles of the feet and legs, then moves slowly upward, to the hips, abdomen, lower back, upper back, neck, and arms. After you have more experience with progressive relaxation, you should be able to relax individual muscle groups—the muscles that support the knee or hip joint, for example, or those that control the joints of the fingers. The following exercise will help get you started:

Progressive Relaxation Exercise

1. Stretch out on the floor with your knees slightly bent; make sure that the small of your back is on the floor so that you do not risk straining the lower back. If you like, support your head with a small pillow.
2. Take a deep breath and tighten the muscles of your feet by clenching your toes.
3. As you relax your feet, exhale. Notice the difference in the way your feet feel.
4. Breathe in again, and tighten the muscles of your calves. Hold the exertion for a few seconds.
5. As you exhale and release your calf muscles, say to yourself, "I feel relaxed."
6. Continue the process, with your knees, thighs, stomach, chest, arms, shoulders, neck, and face. Each time you tighten and release the muscles, feel yourself sink deeper and deeper into a state of relaxation.
7. When you have finished the process, breathe steadily and deeply for 5 minutes, enjoying the sense of relaxation.
8. Repeat the exercise daily.

As you learn more about your body and the way it reacts to stress, you may be able to attain the relaxed state more quickly and directly. For example, you may be working at your desk and notice that your shoulder joints are beginning to ache. To relax them you can tense them further, and then let them relax. When you focus on the warm, relaxed sensation of your shoulder muscles, you may feel your entire body, and spirit, relax as well.

No matter what method of relaxation you choose, try to make relaxing seem to be a release and a joy rather than a chore. These simple hints are meant to help you find peace and avoid frustration:

Plan to relax. When you know a deadline is coming up, or that the week is going to be particularly busy and stressful, try to schedule some time—even just a few minutes—during each day to perform one of the relaxation methods described above or to simply take a walk to relieve the pressure. Chances are, you'll return to the task at hand feeling rejuvenated and better able to focus your attention.

Increase your sense of self-esteem and control. Learning that you have power and control over your internal environment and realizing that you can make successful, positive changes in your physical and mental health will automatically raise your self-esteem and give you a new sense of self-confidence. With patience and dedication, these habits may well become a favorite part of your daily routine.

Remember to laugh. Although it may have become a cliché to say so, laughter truly is one of the best medicines. Humor provides a healthy balance to all the hostility, anxiety, and tension we feel every day. If you can look at the world and yourself with a bit of humor and a touch of whimsy, you'll find that your mind is not as cluttered, your stress is not so great, and your aches and pains are less intrusive and debilitating.

If you learn to meditate at the same time that you begin to improve your diet and exercise habits, you're well on your way to taking control of your life, limiting the damage arthritis can do to your joints, and improving the state of your general health and well-being.

Along with the diet and exercise recommendations given to you in the previous two chapters, we'll take you on a journey to the East, in Chapter 7 to show you how another culture and medical tradition views arthritis and its treatment.

"To wish to be healthy is part of being healthy."

Seneca

7

Acupuncture and Chinese Medicine

Until he was diagnosed two years ago with rheumatoid arthritis, Marlon suffered with achiness and swelling of most of his joints, but managed to resist taking any medication other than aspirin. His wrists, knuckles, and ankles frequently felt warm and puffy, a condition that tended to worsen whenever the weather was rainy or damp. Although he had tried a few natural approaches on his own, he remained frustrated and upset as his condition continued to limit his life. Finally, someone referred him to a local acupuncturist and practitioner of Chinese medicine.

At his first appointment, the acupuncturist asked Marlon many questions, not only about his arthritis, but also about other symptoms and about his sleep patterns, his bowel regularity, fluid intake, and diet. He also asked Marlon about what factors affected his arthritis symptoms, such as whether the pain seemed to move (no), was it sharp or dull (dull), whether warm baths helped (sometimes), and whether rubbing the joints felt good or bad (usually bad). He then diagnosed Marlon has having a "damp bi" syndrome in Chinese medicine, which is one way that painful swelling is described.

The treatment involved putting acupuncture needles near the sites of the swelling, very superficially under the skin. Previously nervous around needles, Marlon was amazed at how little pain was associated with the acupuncture procedure. After a few treatments, the acupuncturist began to concentrate on what he described as the underlying deficiency of spleen energy, which he believed led to Marlon's symptoms. He put needles in points on the legs and abdomen after first warming up the areas with a burning herb called moxa or mugwort. The needle sites bore no anatomical relationship to Marlon's swelling, but were points on channels called meridians, which formed pathways of energy through the body. Marlon also began taking herbs, in a powdered form, twice a day. The herbs were designed to move the "dampness" out of the joints. He was also given a stick of moxa and taught how to use it to warm up his joints every night before bed.

After just a few weeks, Marlon noticed less swelling in the wrists and ankles. As long as he continued to take his herbs and see the acupuncturist twice a month, he felt terrific and no longer needed to take even aspirin to relieve the pain.

Like Marlon, you may find that acupuncture will help to resolve your arthritis pain. It may interest you to know that acupuncture is part of a rich and multilayered approach to health and healing, one that encompasses every aspect of your being—mind, soul, and body.

The Philosophy of Chinese Medicine

At its heart, the Chinese philosophy of health is based on the view that humanity, and each individual human, is part of a larger creation—the universe itself. Each of us is subject to the same laws that govern all of nature. In fact, Chinese medicine refers to the flow of bodily fluid and energy as channels and rivers, and the state of the body as a whole in terms of the natural elements. Don't be surprised if your condition is referred to as "damp" or "dry" or connected to the "water" or "wood" element.

In Chinese medicine, your health is determined by your ability to maintain a balanced and harmonious internal environment. Internal harmony is expressed through the principle of yin-yang, in which two opposing forces have united to create everything in the universe. Yin has connotations of cold, dark, and wet, while yang is bright, warm, and dry. Yin is quiet, static, and inactive while yang is dynamic, active, and expansive.

In humans, parts of the body are ascribed more yin or more yang qualities, as are all physiological processes and disease. To diagnose and treat arthritis, for instance, a Chinese practitioner might focus on determining the yin or the yang nature of the pain as described by the patient.

QI: THE LIFE FORCE

According to Chinese philosophy, all pain is caused when the yin-yang balance in the body is disturbed. Yin-yang becomes disturbed when the flow of energy through the body—energy known as qi (pronounced "chee")—is interrupted or blocked in some way. In Chinese medicine, qi is the energy essential for life. All of your body's functions are manifestations of qi, and your health is determined by your having a sufficient, balanced, and unimpeded flow of qi. Qi ensures bodily function by keeping blood and body fluids circulating to warm the body, fight disease, and protect the body against negative forces from the external environment.

Chinese medicine holds that qi circulates through the body along a continuous circuit of pathways known as meridians. These meridians flow along the surface of the body and through the internal organs. When you are healthy, you have an abundance of qi flowing smoothly through the meridians and organs, which allows your body to function in balance and harmony.

If qi becomes blocked along one of your meridians, however, the organ or tissue meant to be nourished by this energy will not receive enough qi to perform its functions. By locating where in the body qi is blocked, and by releasing it through acupuncture, acupressure, herbs, and exercises, Chinese therapists attempt to restore proper energy flow to the body.

DIAGNOSIS AND TREATMENT OF ARTHRITIS

Like most other branches of natural medicine, Chinese medicine provides no standard diagnostic signs or treatment plans. Instead, you'll be evaluated based on your own unique constitution and energy level. In traditional Chinese medicine, both rheumatoid arthritis and osteoarthritis are know as *bi* (or blockage) syndromes. Qi energy becomes blocked at the joints by cold, damp, heat, or wind or a combination thereof. During the diagnostic procedure, the practitioner of Chinese medicine will attempt to determine your particular pattern of internal disharmony.

Like most of us used to a more mainstream approach to the medical exam, you might find a visit to a Chinese medical office to be a bit on the exotic side. You may pick up the slightly sweet smell of burning moxa, the herb frequently used as part of acupuncture treatments. Even after you sit down with the practitioner, you might be surprised by the course the appointment takes. First, far more time than usual is spent discussing the symptoms that brought you to visit in the first place. The practitioner will ask you to be very specific about your symptoms, asking you when pain occurs, what it feels like (hot or cold, sharp or dull), and what makes it feel better.

She may also ask you more general questions about how you feel or react to heat or cold, dampness or dryness, seasonal variations, and day to night changes in mood and feelings of well-being. Other questions might concern bowel movements, menstruation, and eating and drinking habits. Your answers to these questions will give the doctor an idea of what part of your system might be affecting your joints and what kind of treatment you might require to bring your body back into harmony.

The physical examination that follows may also be a bit different from what you might be used to. A healer trained in Chinese medicine places a great deal of importance on listening to your pulse. In fact, she will feel twelve different pulses, six on each side, and each related to a different organ in the body. The pulses also relate to meridians, the energy pathways through the body, which may result in disease or pain if blocked. Your practitioner may also spend time looking at your tongue. According to the tenets of Chinese medicine, the tongue's coating, color, and shape reveal much about your body. By examining your tongue, the doctor is also attempting to locate where in your body qi flow has been disrupted.

After performing these exams, as well as observing your demeanor, way of moving, and mood, the practitioner will attempt to devise a treatment plan that will help unblock your "stuck" qi and bring your body back into balance. Generally speaking, such a plan will include acupuncture. It might also involve herbal therapy, acupressure and some other massage techniques, and qi-gong exercises. Sometimes practitioners specialize in using one or two of these modalities. And, at the same time, they will help you to find a diet, exercise, and stress-relieving routine to maintain that balance once you've achieved it.

Acupuncture, Acupressure, and Shiatsu

There are over one thousand "acupoints" located throughout the body. These points can be stimulated with needles or with one's own hands to enhance the flow of qi through the body and thus restore health. Your Chinese doctor will show you, on a chart and on your body, exactly where along these channels your difficulty is located.

Acupuncture needles are very long and very thin. Their insertion should be nearly painless, although there is often a mild pin-prick and tingling sensation as the needle makes contact with the qi within the tissue. Often, moxibustion is used to warm and tone the body's qi before the needles are inserted. Moxa consists of special

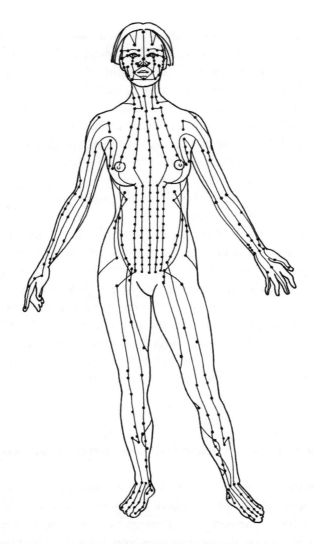

Acupuncture Points

*Traditional Chinese medicine postulates that energy flows
through the body in twelve major pathways called meridians, each
linked to specific internal organs and organ systems. Within
the meridian system, there are over a thousand acupoints that can
be stimulated to enhance the flow of energy.*

herbs derived from the mugwort plant and is gently heated either above or on a specific acupoint.

Acupuncture needles may be inserted to a depth of about a quarter to two inches or more, depending on a variety of factors, including your size and the way that the practitioner wishes to influence the flow of qi. The practitioner always takes care to avoid blood vessels and major organs. The needles are left in place anywhere from a few seconds up to an hour; the average time is about 20 minutes. The type, extent, and location of your arthritis symptoms, as well as the area of blocked qi, will determine how often and for how long you visit your acupuncturist. The average schedule is about once a week for several months, then once a month or so for maintenance.

Acupressure is different from acupuncture in that it uses finger pressure rather than needle insertion to stimulate acupoints. This method is especially helpful for those people who dislike or are afraid of needles, and it has the added comfort of physical, human touch. However, since the meridians and points are below the surface of the skin, it takes a skilled acupressurist to achieve the same level of efficacy as an acupuncturist. In fact, Chinese medical theory holds that a practitioner can transfer her own qi, or energy, to you through her hands, thus helping to heal you with touch. With a little training and guidance, you can learn to stimulate acupoints yourself and perform acupressure at home on your own.

Shiatsu, a massage technique developed in Japan, is another method of stimulating the flow of qi, which in Japan is known as ki (pronounced "key"). The shiatsu therapist may use a combination of fingers, thumbs, elbows, knees, and feet to press acupoints, usually in a rhythmic pattern. She may also stroke your body as well as gently twist your spine and other joints to further relax you.

Acupuncture, acupressure, and shiatsu all have the same goal in mind: to ensure that the life-giving energy is moving unimpeded through your body. Qi-gong exercises, described a little later in this chapter, offer another way to stimulate qi and bring your body back into balance. In addition to these methods, Chinese medicine also uses herbs to nourish the body, mind, and spirit.

Chinese Herbal Medicine

The use of herbs is an essential part of traditional Chinese medicine. They are used to help reorganize the body constituents (qi, blood, and body fluids) within the meridians and the internal organs, as well as help the body to cope with stress and other external forces. In general, Chinese herbal medicine involves using multiple herbs in combinations that have specific effects. Herbs are dispensed and can be used in many different forms, including pills, tinctures (alcohol-based solutions), or capsules. Fresh herbs may also be given. They are to be boiled in water to make teas or used in food.

The doctor of Chinese medicine you visit may suggest certain herbs for you based on your particular problem and constitution. Although it would be counterproductive to attempt to prescribe herbs for you in this text, the following two combinations are known to help relieve arthritis symptoms:

Guan Jie Yan Wan (arthritis combination). This formula is for damp wind pain, that is, for swollen joints. It should not be taken during pregnancy.

Zhui Feng Huo Xue Pian (expel wind and move blood tablet): This is used for painful joints which get better with warmth, are stiff, and might be in the upper part of the body. It is also contraindicated in pregnancy.

Qi-Gong: Chinese Physical Fitness

A fourth form of Chinese therapy is qi-gong, a literal translation of which is "energy exercises." Qi-gong builds qi and helps to move it freely around the body. The exercises work to cultivate inner strength, calm the mind, and help maintain the body's natural state of internal balance and harmony or, if upset, restore the balance.

There are several types of qi-gong. Some exercises are similar to calisthenics or isometric movements, others are like meditative stances, and still others involve the stimulation of acupressure points through massage. Breathing exercises, similar to those described in Chapter 6, are designed to bring the body into a state of relaxation and harmony.

The basic qi-gong posture involves standing with the feet apart, with knees slightly bent, back straight, and the arms held in front of the body. You are then to imagine that you are holding an imaginary "ball of qi" in front of you. This posture is maintained for a few minutes to a half hour, and will improve your circulation, warm your hands, and relax you.

Chinese medicine, with its emphasis on internal harmony and self-care, is appealing to more and more Americans every day. Anxious to avoid the often painful, usually expensive, and almost always futile mainstream treatments for arthritis, millions of men and women find the ultimate goal of Chinese medicine—to bring internal harmony and balance to the body and spirit—both immediately soothing and ultimately motivating.

In Chapter 8 you'll learn about another system of medicine, one developed in India that also looks at health and healing from a holistic and natural perspective.

"The human body is the universe in miniature . . . if our knowledge of our own body could be perfect, we would know the universe."

Mahatma Gandhi

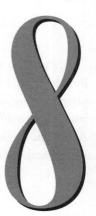

Ayurvedic Medicine

*I*n Sanskrit, the primary language of ancient India, *Ayurveda* means "knowledge of life." Indeed, it is far more than a compendium of medical treatments: It represents a complete philosophy of life and living. Like traditional Chinese medicine, Ayurvedic medicine sees each individual person as an extension of the universe, and health as a state of balance within the body and between the body and the universe. In Ayurveda, as in most holistic forms of health and healing, there is no dividing line between body, mind, and spirit, and disease and pain can be caused by physical, psychological, or spiritual imbalances. Your case of arthritis, in this view, could very well stem from the fact that your life is too filled with stress or that you are unhappy in your relationships with others rather than from misuse or overuse of your joints.

Ayurvedic medicine attempts to treat not just the overt symptoms, but the whole body. It uses a combination of herbal medicine, diet, yoga, and meditation to bring the body back into balance. And as is true in many forms of alternative medicine, the process of diagnosis in Ayurvedic medicine relies far more on a practitioner's powers of observation and questioning than on laboratory tests or imaging techniques.

The Diagnostic Process

If you're like most Americans who are more familiar with Western techniques, it may surprise you that the Ayurvedic practitioner begins by asking you a series of questions about your personal life and habits as well as about your arthritis symptoms in particular. In addition, you may find it strange that he will want to smell and touch your skin during the exam; don't be alarmed, this is a perfectly natural part of the Ayurvedic diagnostic procedure.

The Ayurvedic practitioner will probably begin his examination of you by taking your pulse. In fact, as in Chinese medicine, he will listen to your pulse at twelve separate sites on the wrists—six on the left and six on the right. Measuring the pulses informs the practitioner of the movement of energy—called *prana*—through the body, as well as the general health of each internal organ.

Another important diagnostic tool used in Ayurvedic medicine, as well as in traditional Chinese medicine, is the examination of the tongue. Ayurvedic tradition divides the tongue into areas which reflect the different organs. The coating on the tongue reflects the amount and type of toxins in the organs. For instance, the rear of the tongue corresponds to the lower back and hip area; thus a practitioner may look there first if you come in complaining of low-back pain or arthritic hips.

The practitioner is likely to ask you a great many questions about your medical history, your present symptoms, and your feelings about your personal life and physical condition. The practitioner will take note of not only *what* you say, but also the *way* you say it: The strength and sincerity (or lack of it) of your voice may reflect your willingness to accept responsibility for your own health. Based on the results of these and other examination procedures, an Ayurvedic doctor will attempt to locate your physical and emotional strengths and weaknesses, as delineated by Ayurvedic tenets.

The ABCs of Ayurvedic Philosophy

As you attempt to relate Ayurvedic principles to your arthritis, keep in mind that Ayurveda teaches that all of life—including disease and its symptoms—depends upon learning and developing self-knowledge. In this way, you can look at the pain and limitations arthritis causes you as an opportunity to reexamine your spiritual life and physical state. As you do so, you will learn how to correct any imbalances and thus bring your body back into alignment with the energy of nature and the universe. Later in this chapter, we'll show you some of the ways Ayurvedic therapies may be used to treat arthritis. In the meantime, here is a brief overview of Ayurvedic philosophy.

PRANA (THE LIFE FORCE) AND THE THREE DOSHAS

Known as "qi" in Chinese medicine, the life-providing energy in Ayurveda is called *prana*. Prana is the animating power of life, providing vitality and endurance to each human being. Prana is also considered to be the power behind the healing process. Indeed, Ayurveda teaches that we each have a Divine Healer within us, nourished by prana, that if properly directed can restore health and balance to the body.

Balance is a particularly important theme in Ayurvedic medicine, as it is in traditional Chinese medicine. In this Indian philosophy, balance and harmony are maintained by what is known as the *three doshas*, forces of energy that act upon body substances and organs. When the three doshas are balanced, the body functions harmoniously and in health; when they are out of balance, disease results.

The three doshas are called vata, pitta, and kapha. Vata represents movement; pitta, metabolism and heat; and kapha, structure. Within every cell of the body, these three operating principles must exist in proper balance for health to be maintained. A balance between the doshas will allow your physical, emotional, and intellectual qualities to function with vitality and energy.

According to Ayurvedic tenets, each individual has a specific body type based on one of the three doshas. In essence, one of these qualities—movement, heat, or stability—predominates, helping to form your unique personality and physiology. Your Ayurvedic body type is like a blueprint outlining the innate tendencies built into your system. It helps to explain why you are able to consume lots of salt without suffering any ill effects, while your sister's blood pressure soars when she overloads on sodium. Or why eating plants of the nightshade family, such as eggplant, causes a flare-up of arthritis in your friend, but has no adverse consequences for you. Since a prime goal of Ayurvedic medicine is to prevent disease from occurring in the first place, understanding one's own dosha and practicing a lifestyle designed to maintain dosha balance are essential. By accurately identifying your body type, an Ayurvedic practitioner then is able to diagnose and treat your condition more effectively.

Your body shape, your personality, and many other physical and emotional attributes determine your dosha. Here are short descriptions of each type of dosha as it applies to body type:

Vata (pronounced vah-tah) represents the force of movement within your body. It activates the physical system and is responsible for respiration and blood flow through the body. The seats of vata—the places in the body from which it springs—are the large intestine, pelvic cavity, skin, ears, and thighs. Organs associated with vata include the bones, the brain (especially motor activity), the heart, and the lungs. Vata is the dosha most associated with arthritis and other musculoskeletal problems.

If you are predominately a vata body type, you tend to be rather thin, with prominent features and cool, dry skin. You're inclined to speak rapidly and have an active, creative mind. You probably like to keep irregular hours, and may be prone to feel anxious and worried. Vata's season is autumn—a dry, windy season during which vata people often develop arthritis, constipation, and other diseases of the vata organs.

Pitta dosha governs the metabolic processes of cells. Organs associated with pitta include the blood, the brain (especially memory and learning), hormones, liver, small intestine, and spleen. If you're a pitta body type, you tend to have a medium build, thin hair, and warm, ruddy skin. Pittas are organized, work hard, and have very regular sleeping and eating patterns. Although generally warm and loving, a person with a predominately pitta dosha may also display quick bursts of temper. Pittas tend to suffer from acne, hemorrhoids, and ulcers, and may often feel warm and thirsty. The pitta season is summer, when the heat and bright light may aggravate pitta-related disorders, including rashes, diarrhea, and inflammatory conditions. Pitta arthritis is marked by inflammation and helped by cold applications.

Kapha is responsible for physical strength and stability, and is directly linked to arthritis and other joint diseases. Located in the chest, lungs, and spinal fluid, kapha holds together the structure of the body. Organs associated with kapha include the brain (information storage), joints, lymph, and stomach. If you have a predominantly kapha body type, you tend to be heavyset, with cool, oily skin. Kaphas are often very relaxed and tolerant people, who are slow to anger and have a tendency to procrastinate. They sleep for long hours and may not eat for physical reasons but rather for the emotional pleasure that food brings to them. Kapha types are especially prone to obesity as well as to illnesses of the kapha organs, such as allergies and sinus problems. The kapha season is winter, when the respiratory system is particularly susceptible to colds and congestion. Kapha arthritis is swollen, with dull pain and heavy aching, made worse by cold damp weather.

The Ayurvedic Prescription

All treatment for arthritis—indeed, for all illnesses and imbalances—involves the use of diet and nutrition, herbs, yoga exercises, meditation, massage, and breathing exercises. It is important to remember that Ayurvedic medicine does not treat any condition in isolation;

thus, the whole body must be brought into balance before a specific symptom, like joint pain and inflammation, can be alleviated.

PANCHAKARMA

The first step in your treatment may involve what is called *panchakarma*, which is the process of detoxifying your body of impurities or toxins. Detoxification may consist of induced vomiting, enemas, blood cleansing (by bloodletting and using blood-thinning herbs), and nasal douching—all under the strict and careful supervision of the Ayurvedic practitioner. Yoga, chanting, meditation, and lying in the sun for long periods make up another stage in the cleansing process.

A period of *tonification*, or enhancement, then takes place. During tonification, you'll consume certain herbs and perform particular yoga, meditation, and breathing exercises. At the same time, or perhaps as a next stage in the healing process, you'll spend a great deal of time meditating; this is called *satvajaya* and has as its goal the reduction of psychological and emotional stress, as well as the release of negative emotions and ideas.

Although the above steps are recommended for anyone desiring to attain proper health and balance, those who suffer from arthritis are likely to be prescribed certain specific dietary guidelines, herbal remedies, and yoga exercises designed to bring your *apana vata* back into balance. The apana vata is the subdosha most related to the intestinal tract, and thus the prescription for flushing out impurities that otherwise might collect in joint tissue and hence cause pain and inflammation. However, any Ayurvedic prescription will be quite personal and individual; everyone with arthritis does not have the same physical make-up and thus will not respond to the same treatments.

EATING FOR HEALTH

Dietary measures are particularly personal. The Ayurvedic practitioner will devise an eating plan based on your own specific needs and physiology, designed to help restore your health and alleviate arthritis symptoms. In most cases, a diet to pacify or moderate the apana vata subdosha would include increasing the amount of asparagus, cooked onions, garlic, and okra, while avoiding broccoli, cabbage, as well as vegetables of the nightshade family like eggplant and potatoes. Dried fruits, beans, and certain herbs like coriander seed and saffron are among the other foods that an Ayurvedic prescription for arthritis, back pain, and other musculoskeletal disorders might limit or forbid. However, you should work closely with your practitioner to devise an eating plan that works for you. Supervised fasting, either by abstaining from eating all food or by eating just one food, is a frequent first-line treatment for arthritis and other pain-associated conditions. A fast may include consuming herbs which help to cleanse the body.

YOGA

Yoga exercises are meant to stimulate and stretch your muscles and organs, as well as bring your mind and body into a deeper state of relaxation. There are dozens of yoga techniques and exercises and, in fact, several different schools of yoga, each one with a slightly different philosophy and emphasis. Indeed, the study of yoga in its fullest measure and many levels is a lifetime endeavor, one that, Ayurvedic tradition dictates, leads to true harmony and health.

At the same time, however, yoga poses in and of themselves can be quite helpful in alleviating muscle and joint pain related to arthritis. Yoga poses, performed correctly and practiced regularly, will help you keep your body in balance and the muscles and tendons of your body supple and lithe.

In his book, *Perfect Health*, Deepak Chopra, M.D., describes a three-pronged yoga program that he prescribes to his patients. Called the "Three Dosha Exercises," it starts with an exercise called "The Sun Salutation," which is a complete Ayurvedic exercise that attempts to integrate your whole body, mind, and spirit. It also stretches and strengthens all of the major muscle groups and lubricates the joints while increasing blood flow throughout the body—a perfect tonic for anyone suffering from arthritis.

The Sun Salutation consists of 12 postures that you should perform in a fluid sequence, one following directly after another. It is important that you keep breathing, deeply and regularly, throughout

this exercise. If your joints and muscles are particularly stiff, you'll
want to perform this exercise very slowly, taking care not to strain or
push too hard.

The Sun Salutation (Surya Namaskar)

1. Stand up straight, feet together, the fingers and palms
   together in front of the chest, the fingers pointing upward
   and thumbs touching the chest. This is the traditional Indian
   gesture of respect or homage. If you like, think of the sun
   suffusing your body with energy.
2. As you inhale, raise your arms high and back, the palms
   facing forward. Let your head fall back, bending the spine
   gently backward at the waist.
3. As you exhale, bend forward from the waist and try to
   touch your hands to the floor beside your feet. Come as close
   as you can, but do not strain. Keep your knees slightly bent.
   Try to press your face to your thighs.
4. As you inhale and lift your head, stretch the right leg back
   and go down on your right knee. The left foot stays in position, and if your hands are not already on the floor, then you
   you should place them on either side of your left foot.
5. As you hold your breath, straighten the right leg and bring
   the left leg next to it. Your hands and toes are now supporting your body. From the back of the head to the heels
   should be a straight line. This looks like the "up" position
   in a standard push-up.
6. As you exhale, bend your arms and lower your forehead,
   chest, and knees to the floor. Try to keep your pelvis and
   calves raised by pulling in your abdominal muscles and grip-
   ping your toes tighter.
7. As you inhale, straighten the arms and raise the upper part
   of your body up and back, keeping the pelvis and legs on the
   floor. Your back should form a gentle arc, with your chin
   pointing up. This is known as the Cobra Position.

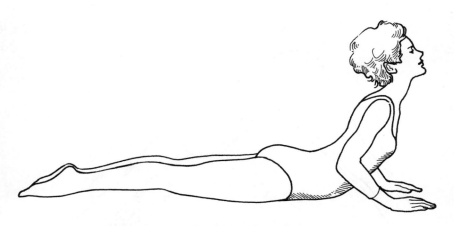

Step 7 - The Cobra Position

*This position works to stretch your hamstrings and lower back.
Make sure that you inhale as you lift and expand your chest forward
and up. Let your upper back widen and lengthen.*

8. As you exhale, raise your pelvis and hips and bring your head between your arms. Your feet should stay flat on the floor, your palms should support your upper body, your back should be straight, and your buttocks should form the highest point. In this Wheelbarrow Pose, you may not be able to keep your feet flat on the floor until you develop a good deal of flexibility.

9. As you inhale, take a long step forward with the right foot, bringing it in line with the hands. At the same time, lower the left knee to the floor and bring the chest up and forward. (This is the same as Position 4, only kneeling with the left knee instead of the right.)

10. As you exhale, assume Position 3 again by bringing the left foot forward beside the right foot, raising the hips, and straightening or nearly straightening the legs.

11. As you inhale, straighten up from the waist and swing your arms high and back, essentially repeating Position 2.

12. As you exhale, lower your arms to the side and stand up straight.

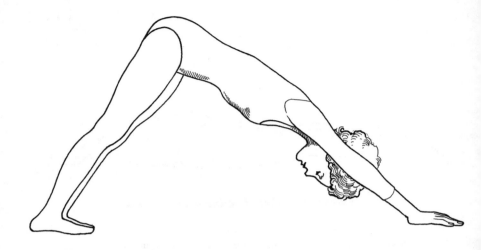

Step 8 - Wheelbarrow Pose

As you perform the Wheelbarrow Pose as described in Step 8 of the Sun Salutation, make sure that you lengthen through the backs of your legs during the stretch, while keeping your head and neck relaxed.

These twelve postures form the Sun Salutation. Once you've done the exercise a few times, it should come naturally to you. Never bounce, strain, or rush. Breathe deeply, feeling energy rush in every time you inhale and tension flee every time you exhale.

If yoga interests you, you should have no trouble finding a class in the city nearest you. A qualified instructor will be able to guide you to the most beneficial poses for your particular condition; if your hips are troubled by arthritis, he may suggest the "seated twisting pose" (*Marichyasana*), which involves a gentle stretch of the spine, neck, and upper body in order to refresh and nourish the lower back and hip area.

Another common prescription for people interested in treating their bodies with Indian healing techniques is called balanced breathing, or *Pranayama*. This exercise involves learning to control and appreciate the act of taking oxygen and prana in and releasing carbon dioxide and other toxins.

To perform a typical exercise, gently close your right nostril with your right thumb, then exhale and inhale once through your left nostril. Now, open the right nostril, and close your left nostril with the middle and fourth fingers and exhale and inhale once with your right nostril. Continue alternating your breath between the two nostrils for five minutes. Remember to remain quiet, begin each breath on the *exhale* and finish on the *inhale*. Breathe naturally, do not feel the need to take deep breaths. You are simply learning to quiet your body and soul while bringing nourishment into your body.

Ayurvedic medicine is an ancient, complex, and multilayered system of health and healing. Its goal—to bring the body back into balance and harmony with nature and its natural state—is one that we should all strive to achieve. The closer we come to that ideal, the less likely we'll be to develop such chronic and ultimately destructive diseases as arthritis. If you are interested in pursuing Ayurvedic medicine in more depth, see our list of resources on page 168. In the meantime, we now look to another system of healing, one that looks to the spinal column and the nervous system that springs from it as the wellspring of health and well-being.

"God heals and
the doctor
takes the fees."

Ben Franklin

Chiropractic and Osteopathy

9

Jules Davidson works as a chef at a large restaurant in New York. After many years of chopping vegetables, kneading bread dough, stirring pots, and working under intense pressure, he began to notice stiffness and pain in his neck and shoulders. His doctor diagnosed arthritis and sent him to an orthopedist. The orthopedist confirmed the diagnosis, further defining the problem as osteoarthritis, or the "wear-and-tear" kind of the disease. The doctor prescribed an anti-inflammatory pain reliever and told him that it was about the only treatment he could suggest. Jules, who hadn't taken a pill in over 60 years, took one look at the prescription then shoved it in his pocket. That afternoon, he made an appointment with a local chiropractor, someone who had treated a waiter at Jules's restaurant for a back problem.

The chiropractor took x-rays of his neck and showed Jules where the vertebrae had become ragged and formed "spurs." She also examined the rest of Jules's back, noting how the spine moved and isolating some areas where Jules felt tenderness in the muscles along the spine. She explained that, over time, the spine had come out of alignment and was thus no longer able to keep the body in balance. This "subluxation," as chiropractors call a misalignment of the spine, led to some irritation of the nerve roots and to the formation of calcium deposits on the vertebrae. She then prescribed a treatment plan that involved Jules coming in twice weekly for six weeks. When told that his Medicare would cover some of the costs, Jules agreed.

During each session, Jules lay face down on an exam table while the chiropractor used a machine that vibrated, loosening the tense, tight muscles in Jules's shoulders and back. After about ten minutes, the chiropractor placed warm packs on his upper shoulders and neck for another ten minutes or so. Finally, she held his upper back, asked him to exhale deeply, then "cracked" his back with a sudden thrust forward. Jules then lay on his back while the chiropractor held his head, rocking it back and forth. When another sudden thrust turned his head, Jules heard a "snapping" noise, after which the chiropractor gave a thrust to the other side. She explained that these were the sounds of once trapped gases escaping from within the joints. Right away, Jules felt that his neck was moving more freely and with less pain.

During subsequent visits, the chiropractor repeated much the same treatments. After a few weeks, she gave Jules a series of exercises to perform every morning and evening to keep his neck more supple and relaxed. He now sees the chiropractor every three weeks and, in between times, feels generally pain-free.

Like Jules, you may have decided that taking nonsteroidal antiinflammatory drugs (NSAIDs) or other medication for your arthritis may do you more harm than good and are searching for a more permanent solution to your problem. Millions of people every year seek help from chiropractors and their cousins in the medical world, osteopaths. Both chiropractors and, to a somewhat lesser extent, osteopaths view spinal manipulation, the adjustment of the vertebrae, as the cornerstone of sound treatment for arthritis and a host of other conditions.

In essence, spinal manipulation therapy is just what it sounds like: treatment of arthritis and other disorders by adjusting the vertebrae of the spine. Twenty-four bones, called vertebrae, make up the spinal column, which surrounds the spinal cord, a sheaf of nerve tissue reaching from the base of the skull to the upper part of the lower back. Between adjoining vertebrae are pairs of spinal nerves, each of which extends to a particular part of the body. Should the vertebrae become misaligned—through trauma, stress, or a chemical imbalance—this places pressure on the nerves or blocks the blood supply to that area. According to those who practice spinal manipulation, the pain of arthritis and its process may be caused or exacerbated by such pressure or blockage. In other words, if the nerves extending from your spine to your knee, for instance, have become blocked, you may feel pain in that joint. Realigning the spine and massaging the soft tissue around the knee will restore proper working order to the joint, or at least release tension and pressure.

Two alternative schools of medicine, chiropractic and osteopathy, consider the spine and the nervous system that springs from it to be the center of all health in the body. Today, more than 94 percent of all manipulative care is delivered by chiropractors, 4 percent by osteopaths, and the remaining 2 percent by general practitioners and orthopedic surgeons. In this chapter, we'll discuss the benefits of chiropractic and osteopathic techniques for arthritis and related problems.

Chiropractic Technique

Chiropractic is a word derived from the Greek *cheir*, meaning "hand," and *praktikis*, meaning "practical." Every culture in recorded history has practiced spinal adjustment, but David Palmer, a self-educated American healer, founded the modern school of chiropractic in 1895. Palmer's first patient was a janitor who had been deaf for almost twenty years. By bringing the man's spine back into alignment through massage and pressure, Palmer restored his hearing. Palmer believed that the janitor had lost his hearing because an injury had damaged his spine, preventing the central nervous system from delivering messages to and from his brain and ear. Palmer also believed that the body has an innate ability to heal itself, an ability controlled by the central nervous system. If the spine becomes misaligned, he believed, then the body can no longer restore balance on its own to any part of the body, including its joints and soft tissues.

Chiropractic therapy centers on restoring proper balance and structure to the spinal column and joints and, by doing so, restoring proper working order to the nervous system that radiates from the spinal cord to the organs and tissues of the body. When the vertebrae are properly aligned and the spine remains flexible, nerve impulses from the brain can travel freely along the spinal cord and to all the organs and tissues of the body.

By keeping the spine in alignment through regular visits to the chiropractor, so the theory holds, you will not only help to soothe the inflammation or tenderness in the joints currently affected by disease, but also protect all of your joints from further injury. And by keeping the nervous system in good working order, you'll be allowing your body to function well as a whole and thus be able to heal itself of most ailments. According to theory, then, chiropractic can be seen as both treatment for injury and pain as well as a method of preventing disease.

CHIROPRACTIC DIAGNOSIS AND TREATMENT

Your evaluation with a chiropractor begins the minute you walk through the office door. The chiropractor will pay as much careful attention to the way you walk, stand, and sit as she will to any x-ray or other diagnostic test. After watching the way you move, the chiropractor will ask you questions about your symptoms and past medical history. In fact, because a chiropractor is not a medical doctor, it is extremely important that you rule out any medical problems that could be causing your arthritis as well as to confirm whether you suffer from wear-and-tear arthritis (osteoarthritis) or one of the inflammatory types (gout, rheumatoid arthritis, lupus, etc.) before you visit a chiropractor. She will ask about any recent injuries that may have caused or exacerbated your arthritis, as well as spend time assessing your work, exercise, and nutritional habits to see how they might be contributing to your problem.

Following this discussion, the chiropractor will administer an orthopedic exam, during which she will pay special attention to the range of movement of your spine and limbs. She may ask you to bend forward, backward, and sideways, and to rotate your spine. She'll also perform a neurological examination, including reflex testing, to assess nerve function in all your joints. Then the chiropractor may feel the spine and various other joints with her hands—a technique known as palpation—to further assess mobility and alignment. Under certain circumstances, x-rays may be required to derive more information or to confirm a diagnosis.

Once your chiropractor decides where your particular misalignment—or *subluxation*, as disturbances in the spine are called in chiropractic—occurs, the chiropractic *adjustment* begins. Depending on what kind of subluxation the chiropractor finds in your spine, she may choose to perform an active manipulation, in which you'll be asked to stretch your body in a certain way yourself, or a passive manipulation, in which the chiropractor assists your movement, helping to stretch the spine past its range of passive movement using her hands. Another process, known as the *high-velocity thrust*, involves the chiropractor placing her hands on a particular vertebral area and then thrusting forward with a certain amount of force and speed. (Jules usually received two or more such thrusts during his treatment sessions.)

The chiropractor chooses an adjustment and technique based on your particular needs and physical constitution. Do not be alarmed if your body makes some cracking or hissing noises: These are signs that the bones are moving and gases within the joints are being released. Although chiropractic should never be painful, you may feel a certain pressure and achiness during, and for a few days following, your first few treatments.

Appointments usually last from 30 to 60 minutes. Most chiropractors will suggest one or two visits a week for a couple of weeks, then one every three weeks for maintenance. Generally speaking, the more entrenched and long-standing your arthritis is, the longer it will take to resolve it. On the other hand, if chiropractic is going to work for you, you should see a substantial improvement in symptoms in about a month to six weeks.

FINDING A QUALIFIED CHIROPRACTOR

Chiropractic now ranks as the second largest primary health care field in the world, with more than 18 million Americans visiting a chiropractor every year. A great majority of these people seek relief from stubborn, chronic pain, including the pain associated with arthritis and other musculoskeletal problems. Today, more than 50,000 chiropractors practice in the United States. Although not medical doctors, chiropractors are among the more highly trained alternative caregivers, requiring at least six years of undergraduate and postgraduate training at colleges accredited by an agency officially recognized by the United States Department of Education. Chiropractors become licensed in all 50 states only after passing rigorous state-controlled exams.

To find a qualified chiropractor, your first step might be to ask your own family doctor. In recent years, chiropractors have been able to form a cordial working relationship with much of the mainstream medical community. Also, feel free to ask your friends and acquaintances for referrals—word of mouth is one of the best ways to find a qualified and caring health professional. Or check with the American Chiropractic Association or the International Chiropractors Association. See *Natural Resources*, page 168 for more information.

Osteopathy: A Holistic Approach

Although this branch of Western medicine remains new to many Americans, osteopathy was founded by a traditional American physician, Andrew Taylor Still, more than 120 years ago. Andrew Still modeled his philosophy of medicine on the theories postulated by the

Greek father of medicine, Hippocrates. Hippocrates believed that the body could cure itself and that a doctor should be trained to study aspects of health rather than symptoms of illness in order to understand and treat disease.

In addition, Dr. Still postulated that the body can function properly only if blood and nerve impulses are allowed to flow throughout the body unimpeded. If your spine or another joint comes out of alignment and blocks blood and nerve flow, disease and pain may result. Furthermore, because the musculoskeletal system is the body's largest energy user, tension or restriction in this system can deplete the rest of the body of its energy and thus result in illness.

Of all the mainstream medical specialties, health professionals consider osteopathy to be the most holistic, tending as it does to treat the whole person rather than one set of symptoms or health concerns. Osteopathic treatment centers on restoring balance and order to the musculoskeletal system—and thus to your whole body—through spinal manipulation. Osteopaths also pay particular attention to diet, exercise, and other habits that may be affecting your health. At the same time, it is important to note that osteopathy is far more mainstream than other forms of alternative treatment. Hence, an osteopath may well prescribe drugs and surgery and may not pay quite as much attention to the holistic side of the arthritis equation as, say, a chiropractor, acupuncturist, or herbalist. For this reason, an osteopath may be a wise choice for you if you are nervous about leaving the mainstream medical world behind completely.

YOUR OSTEOPATHIC EXAM AND TREATMENT

Unlike chiropractors, osteopaths are licensed medical doctors who receive extra training in spinal manipulation and the musculoskeletal system in general. Osteopaths are able to perform extensive diagnostic tests, prescribe drugs, and perform surgery. Although most osteopaths are general practitioners, some may have chosen training in a mainstream specialty, such as gynecology, pediatrics, or surgery.

Your first appointment with an osteopath should be quite similar to one with a mainstream physician, with a few notable exceptions.

First, he will most likely spend more time discussing your general health, your medical history, your symptoms, and your personal habits. Second, he will pay special attention to the way you sit, stand, and walk, and may ask you to perform special exercises to see how your body moves. Asymmetry, a condition in which one side of your body is being held off-center, thus placing stress on that part of the body, is one condition osteopaths attempt to identify. Osteopaths also look for any abnormal increase or decrease to the normal curve of the spine.

Third, the osteopath will probably spend far more time touching your body, particularly your spine and other joints, than a mainstream physician might. He will feel for temperature and texture changes of the skin, areas of muscular tension, tenderness or swelling, and nerve reflexes. In some cases, x-rays or MRI studies may be suggested, depending on what the osteopath finds during the initial examination.

Once the osteopath locates the source of your problem, he will help you work out a treatment plan. In most cases of arthritis, this will involve the following:

Medication and Surgery. Because osteopathy blends conventional with alternative approaches, osteopaths may be more likely than other holistic practitioners to recommend mainstream medical solutions. On the other hand, they are more apt to suggest trying all other approaches at their disposal before attempting more radical solutions such as joint replacement or heavy dosages of pain/inflammation relievers.

Manipulation. Like chiropractors, osteopaths use their hands— and sometimes gentle currents of electricity or ultrasound technology—to release tension from muscles and restore proper alignment to the spine and other joints.

Relaxation Techniques. By prescribing specially designed exercises and visualization techniques (such as those described in Chapter 6), osteopaths help you to maintain your body's structural integrity by preventing stress and tension from disrupting your musculoskeletal system.

Breathing Exercises. Deep breathing exercises are meant to help bring life-enhancing oxygen and other nutrients to all the tissues of the body, as well as to help keep muscles, tendons, and other supportive tissues supple and lithe, and thus the joints more flexible and lithe.

Posture Correction. Borrowing from a variety of bodywork techniques, including some of those described in Chapter 8, Ayurvedic Medicine, osteopaths attempt to correct postural imbalances that may be contributing to your case of arthritis. By teaching you how to use your body in a more efficient and less stressful way, osteopaths hope to help you reduce the stress and tension that may damage the joints and soft tissue in your back and throughout your body.

Nutritional Guidance. Because osteopathy is essentially a holistic approach to health and healing, your osteopath will assess the state of your diet and help you to develop an eating and nutritional plan that will keep you healthy and your joints as free from disease as possible. The plan may include undergoing allergy testing and eliminating nightshade foods such as tomatoes, peppers, and potatoes from your diet.

FINDING A QUALIFIED OSTEOPATH

Today, more than 35,000 osteopaths practice in the United States. The training they receive in the fifteen osteopathic medical colleges blends conventional medical and surgical techniques with osteopathic manipulative techniques. Medical doctors (M.D.s) who are also osteopaths carry the title doctor of osteopathy, or D.O., and are listed in the telephone book under Physicians and Surgeons. See *Natural Resources*, page 168 for information about locating an osteopath through the American Academy of Osteopathy or the American Osteopathic Association.

To a large extent, Western medical traditions form the basis of both chiropractic and osteopathy. In the next chapter, we explore an approach to health and healing that also focuses on the healing powers of touch.

"Most men
die of their cures,
and not of
their disease."

Jean Molière

Healing Touch: Bodywork and Massage

Your skin is one of your largest and most important organs, covering approximately 12 to 19 square feet and weighing between 5 and 8 pounds, depending upon your height and weight. In addition to forming a protective sheath around your muscles, joints, blood vessels, and internal organs, your skin is also an extremely sensitive and animate structure. A piece of skin about an inch in size contains more than 3 million cells, 100 to 300 sweat glands, 3 feet of blood vessels, and more than 50 nerve endings.

It should come as no surprise, then, that when your skin is touched, the feelings generated reach far below the surface into the very depths of your physical and emotional self. And when stronger pressure is applied, your muscles, tendons, ligaments, joints, and even your internal organs receive benefits.

For centuries, healers from virtually every culture around the world have used the power of touch as a method of curing illness and relieving pain. In recent decades, massage and other methods of bodywork using the human hands as instruments of health and healing have finally been gaining in popularity and acceptance across the United States as well.

In this chapter, we discuss some of the ways that bodywork techniques can help to heal the body and bring it closer to the ideal state of balance and integrity we know as health. Performed by expert hands, massage is able to

- help relax the body by calming the nervous system
- soothe tense and cramped muscles and joints
- break up scar tissue and loosen adhesions that may form after injury to joints or during long periods of sedentary activity
- foster healing by stimulating circulation of immune system cells
- trigger the release of endorphins, the body's natural painkillers
- increase blood flow, helping to remove harmful chemical waste products from muscle and nerve tissue
- help reduce swelling and other symptoms of inflammation
- release pent-up, potentially toxic emotions through deep breathing and verbal expression during massage
- bring muscles, bones, joints, connective tissue, and organs back into proper alignment

You have virtually dozens of different bodywork and massage techniques from which to choose. Although the goal of all forms of massage remains to return the body to a balanced, healthy state, each technique is slightly different. Following is a brief overview of several different methods available in the United States today. You can find out even more about them by calling or writing the organizations and agencies listed under "Bodywork and Massage" in *Natural Resources*, page 174.

Please note, however, that if you suffer from severe rheumatoid arthritis in which your joints are currently inflamed and swollen or if osteoarthritis has already caused significant degeneration of bone and joint tissue, you should approach bodywork with great care. Make sure you consult your primary physician or alternative practitioner before you visit a massage or bodywork specialist—especially if the approach you choose involves a great deal of thrusting or joint manipulation. That said, the vast majority of people with arthritis will benefit from being touched and massaged by a trained professional.

Therapeutic Massage

The word *massage* is derived from the Arabic *massa*, which means "to stroke." Therapeutic massage, and its offshoot Swedish massage, involve kneading and stroking the skin and applying pressure on tense muscles. Tapping, clapping, or similar percussive hand movements along the spine and muscles may also be employed. The circulation-boosting aspects of massage often help relieve the pain of arthritis, especially arthritis that has already caused some disability or inactivity. Massage can be a form of "artificial" exercise that helps blood flow, increases the range of motion of limbs, and helps maintain the suppleness of your body's soft tissues—all of which help to keep your joints moving to the best of their ability.

Swedish massage, developed about 150 years ago, is the most popular form of massage in the United States at this time. The technique involves five basic strokes:

Effleurage consists of long, gliding strokes from the neck down to the base of the spine or from the shoulder down to the fingertips. Effleurage is designed to acquaint the therapist with the subject's body, and vice versa.

Petrissage involves gently lifting muscles up and away from the bones, then rolling and squeezing them, again with a gentle pressure. Petrissage is especially useful for people with arthritis because it tends to increase circulation and clear out toxins from muscle, nerve, and joint tissue.

Friction consists of applying deep, circular movement near joints and other bony areas with thumbs and fingertips. Friction breaks down what are known as adhesions. These are knots that result when muscle fibers bind together during the healing process. Breaking down adhesions thus contributes to more flexible muscles and joints. It also helps to induce deep relaxation.

Tapotement is a short chopping stroke applied in several different ways—with the edge of the hand, with the tips of the fingers, or with a closed fist. Tapotement attempts to release tension and cramping. For those in the midst of an arthritis flare-up, this type of stroke might best be avoided, since it can cause an increase in inflammation.

Vibration, or shaking, involves the therapist pressing his or her hands on your back or limbs and rapidly shaking for a few seconds in order to boost circulation and help the muscles to contract more efficiently.

With these five types of stroke, the Swedish therapist will attempt to manipulate all of your muscles, paying special attention to those supporting the joints most affected by disease. In addition to licensed or certified massage therapists, many health professionals now practice massage, including physical therapists, athletic trainers, and nurses.

A visit to a massage therapist typically lasts from 30 to 60 minutes. In most cases, you will be asked to remove your clothing, lie down on a massage table, and drape a sheet over your body. Before he begins the session, the therapist may ask about your medical history and your current emotional and physical state. In some cases, pleasantly scented mineral oils may be used during the massage.

In addition to Western forms of therapeutic massage, of which there are any number of variations, Eastern techniques of massage also flourish. These include *shiatsu* and *acupressure*, both of which developed out of Chinese medical theory.

The Alexander Technique

Posture—the way we hold our bodies as we stand, sit, and move—has a direct effect on the state of our physical and mental health, or so claimed Frederick Mattias Alexander, a turn-of-the-century Australian Shakespearean actor. Plagued by chronic voice loss, Alexander studied the way he spoke by reciting lines in front of a mirror. What he noticed surprised him: Whenever he began to speak, he tended to tense his neck, move his head back and forth, and slightly hunch his back. When he altered these habitual muscular movements, however, he found that his voice returned in full strength.

Based on his own experience, Alexander formulated a theory that the root cause of many disorders—especially those directly connected to the musculoskeletal system such as arthritis—is the muscular tension that results from holding our bodies in the wrong position over many years. He developed a technique by which practitioners could help subjects "unlearn" faulty movements or postures.

The heart of the Alexander technique consists of allowing your spine to slowly stretch upward to its optimal length by releasing the tension in your neck and lifting your head up so that it sits just above the spine. Whenever you move, you should lead with your head, follow with the spine, and let your body lengthen to its full balanced extent. By doing so, the technique helps to expand the spaces inside the body, including the spaces between the bones that form joints.

During a typical Alexander technique session, which can last up to an hour and a half, you might be asked to sit, stand, or lie on a table (fully clothed). The practitioner will then touch your head, neck, and spine, feeling for any tension or muscular compression. Generally, she will move your body into alignment, helping you with words and motion to find your correct posture and thus release your joints from any undue pressure. Eventually, over time, you will learn to hold and move your body in a whole new and, hopefully, pain-free way.

Today, there are about 500 teachers of the Alexander technique nationwide. To be affiliated with the national professional society—the North American Society of Teachers of the Alexander Technique—a practitioner must have had three years and at least 1,600 hours of training.

Physical Therapy

Physical therapists attempt to show individuals how to conserve energy, protect their joints, and treat their symptoms with heat and cold. With the goal of restoring normal—or at least functional—movement, they evaluate movement to recognize and correct abnormal movement. There are a variety of ways that physical therapists can help the people they see. In some cases, treatment will permanently solve the problems, such as occurs with physical therapy after an acute injury or trauma. In other cases, they can help to evaluate and control pain, work to decrease muscle spasm and joint inflammation, and help people learn to use their joints more efficiently and with less stress and strain.

Often, physical therapy is scheduled two or three times a week, especially at the beginning of a program. Physical therapists are highly trained health professionals, having graduated from four or five years of intensive, hands-on experience in a physical therapy program at a university or college. Upon graduation, students receive their B.S. in physical therapy, then must pass a state licensing exam to receive the official title of physical therapist, or P.T.

Myotherapy

A technique developed by Bonnie Prudden, myotherapy is based on the idea that past injuries can result in hidden pockets of pain called "trigger points." Trigger points are tender spots on the body caused by any trauma or injury—emotional or physical—at any age and can be in any part of the body. Trigger points related to arthritis may involve old strains or injuries caused by an accident, by years of poorly performed repetitive movements, or may result from any of a number of emotional wounds and scars. Once activated, trigger points force affected muscles to shorten and remain that way, restricting the range of motion of the joints involved.

When you visit a myotherapist, he or she will first take a medical history and ask you about your symptoms as they stand today. You will then be asked to remove your clothes and put on a gown. Carefully, and using a combination of intuition and training, the therapist will locate your trigger points by gently pressing down upon your back or other body parts. Because trigger points can also "refer" pain to a distant site in the body along predictable patterns, you shouldn't be surprised if your therapist begins to work on your foot or hand first.

Once a trigger point is found, the therapist will apply pressure to the area directly above it using his or her elbow, knuckles, or fingers. Although you may feel some pain along with the pressure, once the pressure is released, the pain often disappears. Because a slight soreness may remain for a day or two as the muscles released try to rewind themselves into their old, tensed positions, the therapist may suggest various stretching exercises and massage techniques you can perform yourself.

In order to receive treatment from a myotherapist, you must be referred by a physician. There are about 200 certified myotherapists practicing in the country today.

Rolfing

This technique, also called *structural integration,* was developed in the 1970s by Ida Rolf, Ph.D., a biochemist. According to Dr. Rolf, pain and disease occur when the body comes out of proper alignment through habitual poor posture and movement. Over time, the fascia (the connective tissue covering muscles and organs) has to compensate and stretch to hold everything in this incorrect and ultimately painful position. As this occurs, the fascia becomes more rigid and solid as adhesions, or scarring, occurs.

In order to return the body to health and balance, Dr. Rolf suggested that the deep connective tissue be manipulated and stretched back into place. As the fascia returns to its natural position, the muscles, joints, blood vessels, and nerves out of alignment slowly work themselves back into place. Finally, the body is remade to conform to its original, balanced design, forming one single vertical line extending from the head and shoulders through the thorax and down into the legs. When this occurs, posture improves, muscles and joints work more easily and with more strength, and self-esteem is elevated.

Rolfing, as this technique is called, is not painless—nor is it completely safe for patients who are experiencing severe arthritis flare-ups. In order to stimulate and realign deep connective tissue, the Rolfer (therapist) must apply some force as he or she massages tissues. It is likely that your first visit to a Rolfer will involve having photos taken of your body in order to assess your posture as you sit and stand. You'll be asked about your medical history, emotional state, and current symptoms of arthritis and other problems. You will then lie down on a table or the floor (fully clothed or in your underclothes) while the Rolfer works through your body, kneading your joints and muscles with his or her fingers, knuckles, or elbows. In this way, the Rolfer intends to reorganize the fascial tissue back into its proper alignment, thereby lifting, lengthening, and balancing the body.

Rolfers receive training at the Rolf Institute in Boulder, Colorado. The course involves two nine-week training sessions, followed by a series of continuing education classes after certification.

Zero Balancing

Zero balancing is a simple, yet powerful hands-on bodywork system, developed by Fritz Frederick Smith, M.D., designed to balance body energy and body structure. Although using a Western scientific base, zero balancing introduces Eastern viewpoints of energy and healing. It works to bring clearer, stronger fields of energy through the body, helping to release tension from both body and mind. This significantly improves physical and mental function, as well as promotes feelings of well-being and optimism in the patient.

A typical zero balancing session takes about 30 minutes. You'll lie on a table, fully clothed, while a practitioner massages and manipulates the joints and soft tissue of the body. The work focuses on the deepest, strongest currents in the body, located in the bones and joints. On one level, a session is designed to improve body function by relieving physical pain and mental tension. On a broader level, because of the clarity of energy flow it induces in the body, zero balancing is especially valuable as a tool to help people through periods of life stress, such as a divorce or death in the family.

Some General Precautions

Although these methods of bodywork and massage are safe for most people, it is important that you follow a few general suggestions before you visit a massage therapist of any kind:

Receive a thorough medical evaluation of your arthritis. As discussed at the beginning of this chapter, there are some cases in which massage or bodywork can do more harm than good, especially if deep massage is performed. Certain types of bone degeneration and inflammation—and the pain they cause—for instance, may worsen with massage. Talk to your doctor or practitioner about your particular problem before making a massage appointment.

Do not receive a massage when you are suffering from a high fever or an infectious or malignant condition. Because massage stimulates blood flow, bacteria, viruses, and even cancer cells may—in certain cases—spread more quickly throughout the body if you undergo massage therapy. Again, talk to your doctor or practitioner if you have any questions.

"Patience is

a bitter plant,

but it has

a sweet fruit."

Old proverb

The Power
of Herbs

11

*A*s foreign as it may seem to those of us accustomed to modern pharmaceuticals, every culture in history has depended on the healing power of herbs. Even modern mainstream medicine is intimately linked to herbal traditions: Trees, shrubs, plants or other natural materials form the basis of approximately 25 percent of all prescription drugs in the United States today. Synthesized versions of natural plants and organic compounds compose another huge segment of the pharmaceutical market. In the rest of the world, herbal medicine is even more heavily used. In Europe, for instance, more than 6 billion U.S. dollars per year are spent on herbal medications.

Although we tend to think of all herbs as plants, an herb is actually any natural substance used for medical treatment. As you'll see in this chapter, herbalists classify two substances—bee venom and shark cartilage—as herbs, and use them quite frequently to treat men and women with arthritis. Also in this chapter, you'll receive an overview of a branch of herbal medicine known as aromatherapy. Dating back to ancient Egypt in about 4500 B.C., aromatherapy is a method of treating illness through the inhalation and external application of essential oils derived from the roots, stems, seeds, and flowers of plants.

Like other forms of alternative therapy, herbal medicine attempts not to cure disease per se, but rather to help the body remain in, or return itself to, the state of balance we know of as health. In attempting to do so, herbalists tend to explore lifestyle and dietary habits with their patients in order to develop a treatment plan far more individualized and personal than most mainstream physicians are able to do.

Although each person who visits an herbalist is likely to emerge with a different prescription (even for the very same complaint), there are some generalities that can be made about possible remedies for arthritis. An herbalist might recommend antispasmodic agents to ease cramping of the muscles; cartilage-building or -repairing substances; anti-inflammatories to soothe inflammation or reduce the inflammatory response; and nervines and tonics that strengthen and restore the nervous system. An aromatherapist might recommend a variety of essential oils for generally the same purposes: to soothe aching joints and to help relax the body and mind.

At a first appointment with an herbalist, you should expect the practitioner to take a complete medical history. Among the most important topics discussed will be the exact nature of your symptoms, the level and type of your physical activity, and any past medical and surgical treatment for arthritis. If the herbalist is a medical doctor or other trained health professional, he or she may also perform a physical exam, concentrating on the joints currently causing you pain. Based on what the herbalist discovers during the exam, he would then prescribe one or more natural medications aimed at strengthening your underlying constitution while alleviating your symptoms. It is highly likely that the herbalist would recommend bodywork, massage, physical therapy, or treatment by a chiropractor or osteopath.

Herbal Medicine: Nature's Pharmacy

In general, herbal medicines work in much the same way as conventional pharmaceutical drugs. Herbs contain a large number of naturally occurring substances that work to alter the body's chemistry in order to return it to its natural state of health. Unlike purified drugs, however, plants and other organic material contain a wide variety of substances and, hence, less of any one particular active chemical. This attribute makes herbs far less potentially toxic to the body than most pharmaceutical products.

Another benefit of natural herbs is that they tend to contain combinations of substances that work together to restore balance to the body with a minimum of side effects. The plant meadowsweet is a good example: It contains compounds similar to the ones used in aspirin that act as anti-inflammatories to treat arthritis and other musculoskeletal ailments. These compounds, called salicylates, often irritate the stomach lining. Unlike commercially prepared aspirin, however, meadowsweet also contains substances that soothe the gastric lining and reduce stomach acidity, thus providing relief from pain while protecting the stomach from irritation. For people with chronic arthritis who have been forced to choose between aching joints and stomachaches, such a treatment can seem like an absolute godsend.

Herbs of all types are available in many forms including:

Whole herbs: Plants or plant parts are dried and either cut or powdered to be used as teas or as cooking herbs.

Capsules and tablets: Increasingly popular with consumers, capsules and tablets allow patients to consume herbs quickly and without tasting them.

Extracts and tinctures: Extracts and tinctures are made by grinding the roots, leaves, and/or flowers of an herb and immersing them in a solution of alcohol and water for a period of time; the alcohol both works to extract the maximum amount of active ingredients from the herb and acts as a preservative.

Poultices and ointments: Ground herbs form the base of external applications that you can place directly on your skin. Poultices are hot packs applied to the skin, made by mixing ground herbs with hot water, placing them in a muslin bag, then applying them to the sore joint or muscle. An ointment is a cream or salve with an herbal base that you can buy in health food stores or through your herbalist.

HERBS FOR TREATING ARTHRITIS

A prescription for an herbal remedy is apt to be quite personal and individual, based on your particular symptoms, habits, and needs. Listed here are some of the herbs prescribed most often for men and women with arthritis:

Alfalfa *(Medicago sativa)*. Also known as lucerne, alfalfa is a nutritious and restorative tonic. Rich in beta-carotene, vitamins C, D, E, and K, and minerals including calcium, potassium, and magnesium, herbalists prescribe it to patients in need of an overall energy boost, as well as to soothe the inflammatory process.

Prescription: You can buy alfalfa in capsule or tea form. A recommended dosage for capsules is 3 to 6 a day, and a cup of tea up to 3 times daily.

Arnica *(Arnica montana)*. Also known as leopard's bane or wolf's bane, arnica is available as an oil or liniment for the treatment of the aches and pains of arthritis. In fact, many commercially prepared liniments contain arnica.

Prescription: Use as an ointment as needed on unbroken skin. If a rash develops, however, stop using it immediately. Never take arnica internally; it is very toxic—the only exception is homeopathically produced arnica as described in Chapter 12.

Bee Venom. Apitherapy is the medicinal use of honeybee products including bee venom, raw honey, pollen, royal jelly, and wax. Like many other forms of natural medicine, apitherapy has been practiced throughout history—ancient references include Hippocrates, Galen, and Paracelsus. Today in the United States, more than 10,000 people—probably many more—currently use this approach to healing.

Apitherapists (beekeepers trained in the use of bee products in the treatment of disease) most often use bee venom in treating arthritis.

Bee venom appears to have anti-inflammatory properties that are most helpful in bringing down swelling and alleviating tenderness in joints.

Prescription: To receive bee venom, you go right to the source—honeybees—and allow one or more to sting you. You do so with the help and guidance of an apitherapist, who has personally raised the honeybees. In some cases, she will apply the bee directly to the sore joint, while in others the spot is a "trigger point," a place elsewhere on the body directly related to the sore joint (perhaps along a meridian as described by Chinese medicine). You may receive two or three stings every other day or up to twenty stings every day depending on the severity of your disease. Needless to say, it is important to know—before you receive your medicinal stings—whether or not you carry an allergy to honey bee stings. Ask your doctor for an allergy test, and always carry a bee sting kit when being treated.

Devil's Claw *(Harpagophytum procubens)*. A traditional African and European remedy for inflammatory conditions like arthritis. This herb acts directly to bring down inflammation (much the way the drug cortisone does) as well as help the body eliminate uric acid, thus reducing the risk of a gout attack.

Prescription: Devil's claw is most commonly available in capsules (to be taken 3 times daily, 2 to 3 capsules each dose) and teas (1 to 2 cups daily).

Feverfew *(Chrysanthemum parthenium)*. Because of this herb's long history of successfully treating fever, migraine, and arthritis, scientists believe that feverfew works in a fashion similar to that of aspirin.

Prescription: Fresh feverfew leaves, steeped in boiling water to make a tea, appear to work best in treating the symptoms of arthritis. Your herbalist may be able to direct you to a source of the herb. Feverfew capsules are also available. Please note that pregnant women should not use feverfew because the herb has stimulatory effects on the womb.

Ginger *(Zingiber officinale)*. Native to southern Asia, the ginger plant, especially its root or underground stem, has been used as a medicine for thousands of years in China. As far as arthritis is concerned, ginger is known to be a strong antioxidant and therefore able to help prevent breakdown of cartilage.

Prescription: Herbalists generally recommend that arthritis patients take about 1 to 2 teaspoons of dry powdered ginger every day. This amount is equivalent to two thirds of an ounce of fresh ginger root—a half-inch slice or so. Ginger is also available in capsules (1 capsule 3 times daily).

Guaiacum (*Guaiacum officinale*). An antirheumatic, anti-inflammatory derived from the heartwood tree, guaiacum is especially useful for hard-to-treat, chronic rheumatoid arthritis.

Prescription: Drink as a tea, made by steeping 1 teaspoonful of the wood chip in a cup of boiling water for 15 minutes, 3 times a day.

Meadowsweet (*Filipendula ulmaria*). Meadowsweet, also known as bridewort and queen of the meadow, is a fragrant herb that contains high amounts of an aspirinlike chemical called salicin. Helpful in relieving pain and fever, meadowsweet does not cause the stomach upset or other side effects common to aspirin.

Prescription: People usually take meadowsweet as a tea, pouring a cup of boiling water onto 1–2 teaspoonsful of the dried herb and leaving it to steep 10 to 15 minutes.

Shark Cartilage. More and more people with osteoarthritis have discovered the benefits of taking shark cartilage supplements. Shark cartilage contains several substances known, collectively, as glycosaminoglycans. One such substance, chondroitin sulfate, helps to stimulate joint repair and improve joint function. In fact, your body appears to be able to absorb the chondroitin sulfate in shark cartilage much more rapidly and efficiently than it can chondroitin sulfate supplements. Nevertheless, as is true for all natural remedies, shark cartilage does not help everyone with osteoarthritis, nor should people expect quick and dramatic changes to their condition. Tracheal cartilage of both cows and chickens has been used successfully and is less costly.

Prescription: You can purchase shark cartilage in capsule form, one capsule to be taken three times a day.

White Willow Bark (*Salix alba*). Also known as salicin willow, this herb works very much like aspirin. It relieves pain, reduces fever, and has anti-inflammatory qualities.

Prescription: White willow products are commonly available in capsules (2 capsules every 3 hours), teas (up to 3 cups daily), and tinctures (1 teaspoon up to 3 times daily).

The Healing Power of Scent

The term *aromatherapy* was coined in 1937 by the French chemist René-Maurice Gattefossé, who badly burned his hand during a laboratory experiment in his family's perfume factory. Knowing that lavender was used in medicine for burns, he plunged his hand into a vat of pure lavender oil used to make perfume. After noticing that his hand healed very quickly, Gattefossé began to explore the healing powers of other essential oils.

Essential oils, composed of the plant's most volatile constituents, are extracted from plants through a process of steam distillation or cold pressing. To derive pure essential oils, no other chemicals or substances should be used during the extraction process since they would disrupt the natural organic composition of plant material. Indeed, each essential oil is made up of several different organic molecules that, working together, give the oil its unique perfume as well as its particular therapeutic qualities.

Like the plants and herbs from which they are extracted, some essential oils are known to have antiviral and antibacterial properties and thus can be used to treat infections such as herpes simplex, skin and bowel infections, and the flu. Perhaps the most common aromatherapy is one that uses oil derived from the eucalyptus plant which, when inhaled, works to restore health to the respiratory system by acting as an antibacterial, antiviral agent as well as helping to loosen phlegm.

Other therapeutic oils ease the anti-inflammatory response in the body, making them especially useful in treating back pain as well as arthritis and similar conditions. In addition, there are a number of oils that have profound effects on the nervous system. Stress overstimulates the sympathetic nervous system and forces the muscles to tense up and, eventually, to shorten, adding to the pain of many arthritis conditions. Certain essential oils, when inhaled, can help to bring the sympathetic nervous system into balance with the parasympathetic nervous system and thus reduce the negative effects stress may have on the musculoskeletal system.

USING AROMATHERAPY

Essential oils are delicate, highly concentrated essences of plants. The quantity of plant material needed to make even a small amount of essential oil is enormous: To make an ounce of lavender oil, for instance, requires about 12 pounds of fresh lavender flowers. Fortunately, only a very small amount of oil is needed to have therapeutic effects.

You can buy essential oils in their pure form or already diluted with another base oil, usually made from olives, soy, or almonds. In addition, herbs which "fix" the scents are added, so that the potency of the mixture is maintained over time. Combining essences with base oils does not change their chemical composition, but will help to reduce their potential toxicity to the skin or internal tissue.

Although it is possible to make your own essential oils with a homemade still, most people choose to purchase prepared oils from health-food stores or mail-order companies. It is important, however, that you make sure that the essential oils you use are just that: essential, meaning that their original chemical compositions were not altered in any way during the extraction process. Make sure that when you buy oils the word "essential" is used on the label and that you buy your oils from a reputable dealer. See *Natural Resources*, page 168, for more information on finding top-quality essential oils.

In general, there are two main ways to use essential oils:

As Inhalants. Simply breathing in the odors and minute particles of plant material will help bring your body back into balance. There are several equally effective methods of inhaling essential oils:

Aroma lamps: Putting a few drops of oil on a light bulb or burning a candle under a cup that has drops of oil in it will volatize the oil into the atmosphere, making your whole environment rich with soothing aroma.

Diffusors: These are mechanical devices that disperse essential oils into the air.

Facial saunas: To use this method, pour boiling water into a bowl, then add a few drops of essential oil. Drape a towel over your head and lean over the bowl so that the towel encloses both head and bowl. The essences are thus absorbed both through the skin and through the membranes of the nasal passages.

As Topical Applications. When prepared properly with base oils, essential oils may be safely and effectively applied directly to the skin. Here are safe methods for applying essential oils:

Bath oils: Adding a few drops of an essential oil to bathwater both adds to the relaxing atmosphere and allows the oils to seep into the skin. Warm baths are also helpful in easing sore, stiff joints.

Massage oils: Oils can be massaged into the face, back, chest, or any part of the body that is feeling pain or stress. A tiny bit of essential oil gently rubbed into the temples each evening can melt away the day's tension. Massage itself, especially when performed by someone trained in the art, is an integral part of any treatment for arthritis as it both releases tension and helps the muscles and joints move back into alignment.

AROMATHERAPY AND ARTHRITIS

The following is a list of essential oils that may help to ease the symptoms of your arthritis, by either reducing the irritating process of inflammation or relieving the stress and tension that trigger and aggravate the pain. Please note that this is a highly subjective list and that many other oils may work just as well, if not better, depending on your own individual constitution and needs. That's why it is important that you visit an herbalist trained in aromatherapy to learn more about how to apply this ancient art to your particular health problem.

Chamomile (*Matricaria chamomilla*). The leaves, flowers, and even roots of this yellow daisylike flower are used in a variety of different ways to treat several kinds of diseases and conditions. Aromatherapists use chamomile oil for its ability to soothe an aggravated nervous system. You can dab a drop or two of chamomile oil on your temples, make a hot compress with chamomile oil and hot water on a terrycloth washcloth and place against an aching joint, or put some oil in a diffuser and inhale it all day long.

Lavender (*Lavandula officinalis*). Probably best known as a perfume, this herb has many valuable medicinal qualities as well. Gently rubbing lavender oils on your temples when you are under particular stress or when the aches and pains of your arthritis are crippling your spirit as well as your muscles is sure to give you a lift.

Coriander (*Coriandrum sativum*). Steam-distilled from the fully ripened but dried fruit of this small plant, coriander oil is used in rubs and massage oil mixtures as a warming pain-easer for arthritis. It should be diluted 1:5 with carrier oil (olive or vegetable oil) before applying directly on the skin.

Eucalyptus Oil (*Eucalyptus* spp.). Although generally used to treat respiratory disorders, eucalyptus may also be applied in ointment form to joints aching from inflammation associated with arthritis. It is especially soothing when mixed with rosemary oil, derived from the rosemary plant.

Rosemary Oil (*Rosmarinus officinalis*). Rosemary oil, distilled from the tops, leaves, and smaller twigs of the rosemary plant, may be used as a massage oil when added to an olive or vegetable carrier oil, or mixed with eucalyptus oil. It may also be inhaled by any of the methods mentioned above (diffuser, aroma lamp, facial sauna). According to herbal tradition, inhaling rosemary oil helps to increase sensitivity to situations, develop a better memory, and strengthen the power of the pineal gland—the gland that secretes melatonin, one of the body's most powerful natural sleep-aids.

Again, although these remedies are generally considered quite safe, it is important that you seek the advice of an herbalist or other health practitioner experienced in the use of herbs for medicinal purposes. Herbs are indeed drugs, and they have the power to cause unwanted effects and side effects if taken carelessly. That said, anyone suffering from a long-term, chronic illness like arthritis is likely to find the use of herbs a welcome substitute or addition to other remedies to relieve pain and stress.

In the next chapter, we introduce another alternative approach to treating arthritis, one that uses natural substances—substances that on face value seem to provoke symptoms of the very condition the treatment is meant to cure—to stimulate the immune system to heal the body. Called homeopathy, it is gaining more attention every day throughout the medical and holistic world.

"Healing is a
matter of time,
but it is sometimes
also a matter
of opportunity."

Hippocrates

12

Like Cures Like: Homeopathy

*M*arjorie Williams, *a 53-year-old woman suffering with rheumatoid arthritis, decided to take a friend's advice and visit a homeopath. At first, the thought of being treated by someone she considered so far out of the mainstream frightened her, but as her flareups became more frequent and severe, she grew desperate. Her friend, who suffered from allergies, had been quite pleased with the results of his treatment, and so she decided to give it a chance.*

Marjorie's appointment with the homeopath surprised her—it was much longer than she had anticipated and it focused not so much on the physical aspect of her condition but upon the way the pain and swelling in her fingers and hips affected her mood. For more than an hour, she described her symptoms in depth, indicating when they tended to occur, how long they lasted, what mood they evoked in her, what made them feel better or worse. She also found herself discussing her personality and in particular her busy schedule filled with volunteer activities. She noticed that the homeopath did not ask very many questions, but instead seemed to watch her posture and gestures very carefully as he took notes on what she said. It came as a pleasant surprise that she did not have to submit x-rays or have other expensive diagnostic tests.

At the end of the interview, the homeopath told Marjorie of the factors that stood out in her particular case of arthritis: the symptoms began as Marjorie entered menopause, she had had heavy periods, and her need to help others was strong. Although Marjorie could not understand how these facts related to her symptoms, she trusted the homeopath's judgment. He prescribed a remedy called Pulsatilla, an herb of the family Ranunculaceae *and also known as windflower, or meadow anemone. He told her that homeopaths had used the remedy since the late nineteenth century to treat arthritis and other conditions. Pulsatilla is particularly effective on people—like Marjorie—who are open, gentle, and compassionate.*

After a few weeks of taking the remedy, Marjorie noticed that her flare-ups were becoming less frequent and severe. Much to her happy surprise, a dry cough that plagued her on and off for some time, but which she had forgotten to mention, also seemed to be alleviated. Although her arthritis has not been "cured," Marjorie feels better than she has in several years and is pleased to notice a sharp decline in her consumption of aspirin and other pain relievers. She knows, too, that she would return to the homeopath should other intransigent health problems arise.

Understanding Homeopathy

In the early nineteenth century, a German scientist named Samuel Hahnemann developed a revolutionary theory of health and medicine. Derived from the Greek work *homoios* (meaning "similar") and *pathos* (meaning "suffering"), homeopathy remains a striking alternative to the way that modern medicine looks at health and disease, particularly chronic conditions such as arthritis. Inside every human, Hahnemann believed, was a "vital force," a life power, that animates and rules the body, keeping it in balance and health. Disease occurs when a disturbance of this vital force takes place. Homeopathy considers symptoms of disease to be the external evidence of the vital force's internal attempts to bring the body back to a state of balance. An aching hip or knee, for instance, might represent the body's effort to release accumulated toxins and waste products from the muscles.

Furthermore, Samuel Hahnemann was a deeply spiritual man who believed that a physician's role should be to help a patient's own body heal itself, that true healing could not take place by simply administering drugs that would, in essence, override the body's natural processes. To a homeopath, a "disease" consists of the symptoms produced by the body in its own efforts to heal itself. To help the body achieve that goal—to strengthen its vital force against an illness—a homeopath administers remedies designed to match these symptoms, not to alleviate them as Western medicine attempts to do. This principle is known as Hahnemann's *Law of Similars*, or "like cures like." By making symptoms worse, a remedy attempts to strengthen the body's own power to heal itself. In fact, according to homeopathic theory, any therapy that attempts to suppress the free flow of symptoms—including the use of painkillers—will actually prolong the underlying disturbance since it prevents the body from being able to heal itself.

Another theory of homeopathic medicine is known as the *Law of Infinitesimals*. First developed by Hahnemann in order to reduce the side effects of often potentially toxic chemicals, this theory states that the smaller the dose of medicine, the greater its potency and its effect on the body's vital force. Homeopathic remedies are extracts derived by soaking plant, animal, mineral, or other biological material in alcohol or water to form what homeopaths call the "mother tincture." This tincture is again diluted with alcohol in ratios of one part tincture to 10 or 100 parts of alcohol or water shaken vigorously, then diluted again.

This process of shaking and diluting, repeated several times, is known as "succussion." Many researchers believe that through succussion the vital energy of a substance is transferred to the tincture. Therefore, the more times the solution is passed through succussion, the more potent the remedy, even though there appears to be no trace of the original herb or mineral left. Finally, the resulting solution is added to tablets, usually made of sucrose and lactose.

As you know from reading about Marjorie Williams's experience, homepaths write prescriptions only after they carefully evaluate a patient's particular set of symptoms and physical and emotional make-up. Indeed, a session with a homeopath may be a unique experience for those of us accustomed to Western medicine's approach to diagnosis and treatment. Generally speaking, a homeopath will spend much more time talking to a patient about symptoms and lifestyle factors, and look more carefully at her demeanor, personality, and coloring, than would a mainstream physician.

According to homeopathic tenets, mental and emotional disturbances are more serious than physical illnesses, primarily because they can themselves cause physical disease. High stress levels and the emotions they provoke (such as anger, anxiety, and irritability) may cause or exacerbate the pain of arthritis. A homeopath will spend a great deal of time talking to you about stress and your ability to cope with it before she prescribes a remedy.

In fact, the way a homeopath treats chronic conditions like arthritis pain depends entirely on an individual's particular pattern of symptoms: not everyone with inflammation of the finger joints, for instance, experiences the same kind of pain at the same time or in exactly the same place, or for the same reasons. While a conventional, mainstream physician would probably offer roughly the same treatment to almost everyone (usually a combination of painkillers, exercise, or surgery), a homeopath recognizes several different symptom patterns and has corresponding remedies for each one. The homeopath then matches the patient's symptoms with the pattern of symptoms produced by a remedy. The more closely the remedy matches the total pattern of the patient, the more effective the remedy will be.

Furthermore, the symptoms that first bring someone to the doctor (called *common symptoms* in homeopathy) are rarely the most important symptoms when it comes to selecting a remedy. Instead, homeopaths give *general symptoms*, which include the patient's state of mind and mood, more weight in determining a treatment. Other symptoms, called *particular symptoms*, are those that pertain to any given organ or structure of the body (muscle pain, for instance). They, too, are less important than the general symptoms. Most important of all are what homeopaths call *strange, rare, and peculiar*; as their name implies, they are symptoms that are completely unique to the individual describing them. A man who says that his knees feel as if they are locked in place and a woman who feels as if her fingers are on fire are examples of two people with strange, rare, and peculiar symptoms. Even if each of them also has been diagnosed with arthritis, they would probably be given different remedies by a homeopath.

One more important aspect of homeopathy is the *Law of Cure*, which postulates that symptoms disappear in the reverse order of appearance. In other words, the last symptoms to appear will be the first to disappear with treatment. If someone has had many health problems in his life, he may find that symptoms of past problems reappear as homeopathic treatment continues. Someone who comes to a homeopath with arthritis, for instance, may find that she briefly develops symptoms of bronchitis, a previous illness. Marjorie found that her cough, due to an unknown underlying problem, briefly emerged but then disappeared. Slowly but surely, working backward in time, the homeopathic remedy or remedies will restore strength to the vital force and balance to the internal environment.

Arthritis and Homeopathy

Treatment is dependent on symptoms, and any of the several hundred homeopathic remedies described in Hahnemann's *Materia Medica Pura*, upon which modern homeopathy is based, might be

prescribed for a person with arthritis—either osteoarthritis or rheumatoid arthritis. In addition, a homeopath would work with someone to
resolve the underlying physical and emotional problems that contribute to the pain—problems that are uniquely personal and impos-
sible to categorize or elucidate. That said, there are some general
recommendations for homeopathic remedies that might apply to you:

Arsenicum album (*arsenic trioxide, white oxide of arsenic*). In
its crude form, arsenic is a deadly poison: when applied topically, it
can literally corrode skin tissue; when ingested, it damages blood vessels and ultimately leads to organ damage throughout the body. However, in the right form and amount, arsenic is known to be a treatment
for several different illnesses—and has been known as such since
physicians in ancient Greece and Rome started using it. Samuel Hahnemann introduced arsenic to homeopathy in 1828, and it has been
used as a remedy ever since.

Homeopaths generally prescribe arsenicum album to those people
whose symptoms tend to be worse at night than in the morning,
improve with heat and warm drinks, and include anxiety and fear.

Aurum metallicum (*metallic gold*). Similar to the gold compounds used to treat arthritis in mainstream medicine, aurum metallicum is a remedy for a variety of disturbances. Homeopathic gold
comes in a fine brown powder which is prepared by a process called
trituration. Trituration, which involves grinding down the powder and
diluting it with milk sugars, is necessary because gold is not soluble in
water or alcohol.

Typically, homeopaths prescribe aurum metallicum to arthritis
patients who complain that the pain in their fingers or limbs feels
worse from sunset to sunrise, is least problematic in the morning, and
gets better during the day.

Bryonia alba (*wild bryony, wild hops*). Bryonia, which is
derived from a climbing vine known as Cucurbitaceae, is one of the
most effective homeopathic remedies for rheumatic conditions. It
acts especially on fibrous tissues, including ligaments and tendons,
as well as nerves. The illnesses usually associated with bryonia

are more likely to occur in warm, damp climates.

A homeopath is most likely to suggest bryonia to an individual who seems sluggish and dull of mind, whose symptoms improve with exposure to cool, fresh air and worsen with movement and touch. Rest and a diet consisting mostly of cold foods may also be recommended.

Calcarea carbonica (*Calcarea ostrearum, oystershell*). Derived from the pure white portion of oyster shells, this homeopathic remedy has as its primary component the mineral calcium. The fifth most abundant element in the body, calcium is essential to the body's formation and repair of bone tissue. Calcarea carbonica, therefore, is especially useful for those people suffering from osteoarthritis.

A person for whom this remedy would be most helpful would have symptoms that improved in a dry, warm climate and worsened in the cold and with any type of exertion. Generally speaking, the calcarea patient tends to have pale skin and a plump figure, among other qualities.

Pulsatilla (*windflower, meadow anemone*). This remedy derives from the perennial herb known as *Pulsatilla nigricans*; it is prepared from the whole fresh plant when it is in flower. In addition to its use as a remedy for arthritis, it is also known to help in eye disease, uterine disorders, and menstrual cramping.

For those with arthritis symptoms, a homeopath is most likely to prescribe pulsatilla to someone who, like Marjorie, is warm and compassionate, complains about the heat, and (if female) has associated menstrual problems. Symptoms tend to worsen with heat and rich food, and improve with open air and cold applications.

Rhus toxicodendron (*poison ivy*). Derived from a plant with which campers, hikers, and adventurous children are all too familiar, this homeopathic remedy was first used by a French physician in 1798. It affects the skin, mucous membranes, and, of special importance to those with arthritis, fibrous tissue including joints, tendons, and sheaths.

People who do best with *Rhus tox.*, as it is known, tend to be anxious and despondent and have symptoms that improve with warmth and warm, dry weather. Other common traits of *Rhus tox.* include frequent rashes, dryness of the mouth and throat, and a dry cough.

It is important to keep in mind that along with these remedies are a host of others that a homeopath may prescribe for your particular symptoms and underlying conditions. As is true for most other forms of holistic medicine, homeopathy is completely individualistic in its diagnostic and prescriptive methods. That means that the success you experience with this type of medicine depends largely upon the homeopath you choose. It will be his powers of observation and judgment that determine the remedies to be prescribed, and it will be he who will monitor your condition over the course of several months. For this reason, we recommend that you receive a referral—from a friend or from one of the associations listed in *Natural Resources*, page 168—before visiting a practitioner.

So far, you've read about eight different holistic medical disciplines that may be appropriate to help alleviate your arthritic problems. No doubt you have many questions, especially if this is your first exposure to information about one or all of these alternatives. In the next chapter, we address some of the most common concerns and issues raised by people new to natural medicine. Even if you're familiar with the tenets we've described, you may learn something useful about how you can successfully apply them to your own case of arthritis.

"That true
bible . . . the
human body."

Andreas Vesalius

Developing an
Alternative Plan

13

....

*Y*ou've now had a chance to read about the many natural
alternatives to drug therapy available to help you cope with arthritis—both its process and its symptoms. These options all have a common goal: to bring your body into a natural state of balance so that
your musculoskeletal system can function properly. They each
attempt to teach your body to heal itself, with help only from natural
substances, human touch, and common sense.

There are some significant differences in philosophy between various alternatives, however, and deciding which alternative is best for you is
a highly personal decision, one that may involve investigating several different options before committing to a particular treatment plan. The following ideas about why and how to choose and use an alternative health
care method may help you make some decisions about your next step:

Use holistic medicine as a preventive tool. It is never too early to make sure that your body is in balance by following a holistic approach to health, especially when it comes to a chronic, generally slowly progressive disease like arthritis. The sooner you take control of your health, the more likely you'll be able to both prevent further degeneration of your joints and avoid stress-related chronic strains and pains over the long term.

Invest in some bibliotherapy. A fancy name for learning through reading, bibliotherapy will help you gain a more thorough understanding of the various philosophies of health and disease before you decide how you would like to address your particular medical problem. In *Natural Resources*, page 168, you'll find a list of the most relevant books on arthritis and natural medicine from which you can choose should you decide to further expand your knowledge of your condition.

Work with a mainstream physician who is willing to explore options with you. As we move toward the twenty-first century, more and more medicine is bound to include the best of both mainstream and alternative options. If your physician is willing to learn, but does not know much about these options, you can share your resources, and this book, with him or her. If you are currently being treated by a physician who is not open to other philosophies and methods, you may want to consider choosing another doctor more sympathetic with your needs.

Live well and in harmony with the universe. If after you've read this book, you decide not to pursue an alternative form of medical care, you still should attempt to open your heart and mind to the natural flow of energy, within and outside of your body. Think about the way you live your life on a day-to-day basis: Is it truly healthy? Does the food you eat nourish your spirit and your body, or do you end up feeling bloated and grouchy? Are you ever able to relax completely, or do you feel under constant pressure? Are your muscles, tendons, and bones strong and supple, or do you often feel stiff, sore, and achy after performing the mildest of exercise? Consider the way you feel every day, and if you think you could feel better, work to make small, incremental changes in your daily habits—even if you decide to forgo a comprehensive natural medicine approach to arthritis.

The rest of this chapter is devoted to answering some of the questions my arthritis patients have asked me, not only about their specific problem, but also about the various treatment options described in this book. We hope that the answers provided address some of your own questions and concerns.

Arthritis and Alternative Medicine

Q. I've suffered from rheumatoid arthritis (RA) since childhood. So far, the pain medication and anti-inflammatories have allowed me to manage my condition, and I have relatively few flare-ups during any given year. But I saw my grandmother, who also had RA, decline rapidly when she hit her 60s. Will natural medicine help me avoid the same fate?

A. It's quite possible. Because both rheumatoid arthritis and osteoarthritis tend to be progressive diseases, the more you can do now to limit the damage, the better off your later years will be. Any number of the alternative options offered in this book will help you get started. Check your diet to make sure you're not eating foods that trigger or exacerbate arthritis flare-ups. Make sure you're exercising your joints every day, taking them at least through their full ranges of motion on a regular basis. Are your stress levels in the manageable range, or could you use some help in releasing tension from your body and soul? Without doubt, the more of these practical issues you deal with now, the better off you'll be in the long run. In addition, receiving herbal, bodywork, and other natural treatments for your arthritis today will help you avoid the side effects—both physical and emotional—that occur with long-term use of anti-inflammatory and pain-relief medication.

Q. I've lived to the age of 64 using mainstream medicine to help me survive a heart attack and a car accident. I know that I'm alive today thanks to the high-tech medical care I received at the hospital after those events. Now that my doctor diagnosed me with osteoarthritis—which has attacked my left hip rather badly—I want to explore alternatives, but I don't want to give up on what has worked for me in the past.

A. There is no doubt that modern medical technology saves lives and can help a patient during an acute crisis. Nevertheless, the effectiveness of modern medicine has its limits, including its typical lack of attention to prevention and its frequent inability to address the root causes of chronic, lifestyle-based conditions like arthritis. Fortunately, we are living in a time when high-tech medicine and its holistic counterparts are learning to work in cooperation with one another. Osteopathy is a particularly good example. Osteopaths are medical doctors, with access to, and an affinity for, mainstream medical techniques. Many chiropractors, acupuncturists, and other alternative practitioners also have medical degrees and working relationships with mainstream doctors and health care facilities. Therefore, you'll still have access to the lifesaving (or pain-reducing) diagnostic techniques and medical therapies you feel work for you while investigating holistic options.

A Medical Overview

Q. My grandmother had rheumatoid arthritis and now so do I. Could something like this be hereditary? Should I worry about my kids?

A. "Nature vs. nurture" is one of the oldest conundrums in medicine. It could be that you've inherited an overactive immune system or muscle/joint weakness and passed those traits along to your children. What is a more likely scenario, and ultimately a more empowering one, is that you inherited certain unhealthy habits, including overeating, underexercising, smoking cigarettes, or leading a life filled with too much stress. As for your own children, it's never too early to instill healthy habits that will help your children maintain proper balance and health. By instilling proper diet and exercise habits in your children from a very young age, you could help prevent them from developing musculoskeletal problems later in life. At the very least, you'll help them to limit the damage that is done should the disease strike despite your best efforts.

Q. I've been working as a seamstress for a fashion designer for about eight months. I love my job, but my neck and upper back are under constant strain. With exercise, I'm able to work out most of the stiffness, but I'm afraid that, over time and as I get older, the pain will become entrenched. Could arthritis develop? What can I do to keep my job but protect myself from injury?

A. You're right to start thinking about a solution now, before arthritis does too much damage to your muscles and joints. The first step you might want to take is to consult a specialist in ergonomics: a person trained in making the workplace safe and efficient. She would work with you to make sure that your sewing machine is in an optimal position, that you hold your fingers, wrists, and shoulders properly as you sew, and that your seat level is correct. All of these measures will help protect you from injury as you work.

Q. What are over-the-counter arthritis drugs? Do they work?

A. Man-made drugs, also called pharmaceuticals, are not necessarily considered "bad for you"; in fact, some drugs may be veritable lifesavers under certain circumstances. Self-described "arthritis medications" available over-the-counter are usually simply stronger versions of aspirin, acetaminophen, or ibuprofen. They may or may not be effective in alleviating your particular pain and inflammation. The thing to remember is that all pharmaceuticals—over-the-counter and prescription—usually focus on alleviating symptoms, not on addressing underlying problems. They also tend to take over body functions rather than help the body to work properly on its own. Finally, drugs often produce unpleasant side effects that, in essence, only add to the state of imbalance that caused the original symptoms to occur. Choosing more natural approaches, such as dietary measures, exercise, and herbal remedies, that attempt to

restore the body to proper working order while producing a minimum of side effects is often a much safer alternative.

Choosing an Alternative

Q. I want a homeopath to treat my arthritis. My mainstream
physician, who admits to being able to offer me few solutions, objects
strongly. What should I do?

A. That's a delicate question without an easy answer. Many reputable and highly qualified mainstream physicians find it difficult to
accept the tenets of homeopathy and other forms of alternative health
care because many haven't been "proven" according to strict mainstream criteria. But as more studies confirm that mainstream medicine
can do little for people with arthritis, more mainstream physicians are
willing to explore options with their patients. If your doctor refuses,
then I might suggest that you find a new mainstream physician, one
who is more willing to explore other treatment options with you.

Q. I've been suffering with joint pain—especially in my spine and
shoulders—almost constantly for almost a year. At least once or twice
a week, I take a muscle relaxant so that I can sleep and I practically
live on ibuprofen and aspirin. Are there alternative therapies that will
allow me to quit taking these drugs?

A. All forms of alternative medicine have at least one goal in common: to allow the body to return to its natural state of balance and
health. Medications like aspirin and ibuprofen, on the other hand,
work by masking symptoms like pain and discomfort, symptoms that
are meant to be warning signs that something has gone wrong in the
body. Pain medication can be enormously helpful in reducing the often
agonizing pain of an acute arthritis flare-up. However, these drugs
may end up doing you more harm than good if you don't address the
underlying cause of your disease and use all of the methods available—including diet and exercise—to help relieve symptoms. It makes
sense for you to begin to look for other solutions rather than simply

depend on these drugs to make your life bearable.

Q. I'm very interested in finding a healthy alternative to drugs and surgery and have been reading about the many different options, particularly traditional Chinese medicine. But I've never been a religious person and the emphasis on a spiritual force that helps us heal bothers me.

A. Spirituality is a belief that we are connected to and dependent upon something outside of ourselves, whether that something is nature, each other, or the unknown. It is important to distinguish this from religion, which is a specific belief system that defines and explains that connection. Although Eastern healing systems stem from philosophical and religious beliefs, it is perfectly possible to derive benefits from these systems without subscribing directly to the philosophy. What is important is a belief that you have the power to control your health and your future, and that you can do this by altering the external world (by diet, stopping smoking, exercising, and changing stressful situations) and the internal world (by not holding onto emotions, by learning to relax, to love and to play, and by being hopeful and having positive thoughts). Perhaps, through this process, you'll also find a new way to address spirituality in your life.

The Food Link

Q. I've been dieting since my doctor told me that the excess weight I'm carrying is part of the reason why my knees and ankles hurt so much whenever I have a rheumatoid arthritis flare-up. I've cut out almost all fat from my diet, mostly because I'm using so many of the fat-free products now available, but I haven't been able to lose any weight. In fact, I think I've gained some. What am I doing wrong?

A. You may be eating as many calories and as much sugar as you have in the past—or maybe more. Although consuming too much fat, particularly saturated fat like butter and animal fat, is the major cause of weight gain, the fact is that eating too much food of any kind—fat-free or not—will put on the pounds, too. Indeed, every time you eat more calories than you burn off, you gain some weight. Make sure you're not overloading on empty calories—like those that make up fat-free chocolate cake—at the expense of lower-calorie, healthier foods like grains and fresh fruits and vegetables.

Q. I consume quite a lot of diet soda. Could the preservatives and additives in the soda be contributing to my arthritis?

A. It's possible that a sensitivity to those substances could be irritating your joints and muscle tissue. However, I would look at more likely sources of the problem first, such as how much you exercise, the work you perform on a daily basis, and even more likely food culprits, like those of the nightshade family.

Q. I love to eat fish and hear that it's a good source of protein and pretty low in fat. Am I right?

A. As long as you don't cook your fish in fat or load it with heavy cream sauces or dressings (like tartar sauce), you've made an excellent choice for your general health and for any weight loss efforts you've embarked upon. Not only does fish tend to have less fat than meat does, but the fat that is in fish contains a special substance, omega-3 fatty acids. These fatty acids, found in salmon, mackerel, tuna, herring, and anchovies, reduce the aches and pains associated with inflammation.

Q. Is it possible to cure arthritis through diet alone?

A. Because the causes of arthritis—indeed, of any chronic disease—are varied and complex, it is unlikely that changing just one aspect of your life will permanently alleviate your problems. Keeping yourself at a normal weight and providing your body with all the raw materials it needs to build and maintain muscle and bone will, of course, help you stay balanced and centered.

Bringing your body into a true state of harmony involves not only addressing nutritional deficiencies or excesses, but also examining your emotional and spiritual state and working to find inner peace. That's why a holistic approach, as embodied in traditional Chinese or Indian medicine, is a good choice for many people suffering from arthritis.

Exercise and Rest

Q. I know that exercise is an important part of any treatment for arthritis, but I also know that exercise can cause injuries. I also have high blood pressure. Should I exercise or not?

A. Before you start any exercise program, get your doctor's permission. If your joints are severely damaged or your blood pressure dangerously high, he or she may recommend very mild and short periods of exercise for a number of weeks—say, walking at a slow pace for ten minutes—until you build up some cardiovascular and muscular endurance. Your doctor will probably recommend that you have a stress test performed at various intervals to test the strength of your heart and may ask you to see a physical therapist for advice. However, starting and sticking with an exercise plan will definitely increase your mobility, improve your cardiovascular health, and raise your general sense of self-esteem and confidence over the long term.

Q. I love to play tennis, and it's about the only exercise I get on a regular basis. But whenever I do a backhand down the line, I seem to wrench my elbow. My doctor says it's tennis elbow. Is that the same thing as arthritis? Is there anything I can do about it?

A. Ask a trained sports therapist to work with you to help identify your problem. It could be related to arthritis or it could be a sports injury. The root of the problem might be your form: You may be hitting the ball improperly, thereby straining your muscles. Or you might need to strengthen your shoulder and wrist muscles through weight training or other exercises before they are strong enough to properly execute the stroke.

Releasing Pain through Relaxation

Q. I have a high-pressured job as a salesperson at a department store and typically work 12 to 14 hours a day. I know I need to relieve some stress. Ever since I started this job my gout, which used to come and go only infrequently and mildly, has been attacking more often and more severely. But it seems that every time I try to relax, I only end up getting more tense. How do I resolve this frustrating dilemma?

A. Take a look at the way you're trying to relax. Although we tend to relate inactivity with relaxation, many people find that activities that stimulate their minds and/or bodies—such as exercising or working at a hobby—are more helpful in relieving stress than sedentary, passive activities like watching television or trying to force yourself to nap.

At the same time, it is important for your general health, as well as for the health of your joints, to try to slow down and quiet your mind on a regular basis. A meditation technique like visualization, which does engage the imagination, may be one way for you to both relax and get in closer touch with what makes you such a driven and tense person in the first place.

You should also take a look at the physical demands on your joints that your job makes. Standing all day long greeting customers may be placing a great deal of strain on your ankles and knees, just the joints that your gout is most likely to attack. That's not to say you should switch careers, but you may want to make some adjustments, especially during a flare-up.

Is there some way you could sit down for a bit, say, approximately ten minutes every hour? Talk to your practitioner and then your boss to see how you can avoid situations that drain your energy and sap your health.

Q. Every night after I get home from work, I spend five or ten minutes writing down everything that I have to do the next day and all the things that are bothering me. I think it helps me relax, but my wife claims that it only makes my problems seem more important than they are. Who's right?

A. More than likely, you are. A study at Pennsylvania State University showed that people were able to reduce their anxiety levels by setting aside a "worry period" every day. If they started to fret about their problems or future tasks at other times in the day, they forced themselves to postpone it until that period. The organization such a system provided gave the subjects a feeling of control that calmed them down. I'd say you were on the right track.

Acupuncture and Chinese Medicine

Q. I'm deadly afraid of needles, but I'm ready to try anything that might help relieve my arthritis pain. My brother goes to a traditional Chinese doctor whom he trusts. Should I put my fears aside and go, too?

A. Before you decide upon acupuncture, talk to the Chinese health care practitioner about your anxiety over needles. There are other options within Chinese medicine, including acupressure, massage, herbal treatments, and dietary measures, that you might want to consider.

Q. I have been to an acupuncturist who used a lot of needles, and left them in for a long time. My friend went to another acupuncturist who used very few needles, and just stuck them in and out. What is the difference?

A. There are several different systems of acupuncture being practiced in the United States, depending on the acupuncturist's training. Chinese style, as you experienced, tends to use several needles which are retained. Japanese style uses a more gentle stimulation and fewer needles, and French style, favored by many physician-acupuncturists, is somewhere in between. English Five Element style tends to focus on the relationship of emotions to the symptoms, while some others tend to address specific physical symptoms. It is best to discuss the system with the acupuncturist prior to or at the first appointment.

Q. I would try acupuncture, but I'm worried about AIDS. Are acupuncture needles risky?

A. In this era of AIDS awareness, it is highly likely that your acupuncturist is using disposable, single-use acupuncture needles. In addition, all licensed acupuncturists are required to take clean-needle training as part of their examination for licensure. Even so, it is important to ask your prospective acupuncturist if he or she uses disposable needles.

Ayurvedic Medicine

Q. Ayurvedic medicine seems very elaborate and multilayered. How much do I have to understand before I can start to heal my arthritis, relieve my pain, and help to bring my body back into balance before I do further damage?

A. Learning about your body from an Ayurvedic perspective is a process, one that may take many years, indeed a lifetime, to go through. An Ayurvedic practitioner will guide you through that process while providing you with practical information about proper diet, exercise, herbal medicine, and meditation techniques. If you follow this advice, you should see positive change in the state of your health relatively quickly, probably within a period of several weeks, depending on your condition.

Q. I don't have a lot of time during the day to both exercise and meditate. Can I do both at the same time with yoga?

A. Yes. Yoga is used as both a form of exercise and a method of attaining a higher state of consciousness through proper breathing and meditation. The beauty of yoga exercise lies in its ability to bring the body into balance through quiet, powerful stretching and bring the spirit into a more relaxed state through focused breathing and, sometimes, creative visualization.

Chiropractic and Osteopathy

Q. Can spinal manipulation, with all of the cracking and pressing it involves, end up hurting rather than healing joints?

A. When performed by a trained professional, spinal manipulation will not damage the joints or muscles. In fact, the idea is to bring your spine and other joints back into proper alignment and thus relieve aches and pains that occur when your body is out of position. And keep in mind that the cracking and popping you hear occur when gases are released from inside the joints when they are moved. This is a harmless, toxin-releasing process.

Q. I've been seeing a chiropractor to help relieve the pain in my shoulders and elbows thought to be caused by arthritis. Recently, my medical doctor told me that my blood pressure, which had been on the high side, is now normal. Could there be a connection?

A. Absolutely. Depending on where on the spine your chiropractor is working to alleviate your symptoms, therapy may be helping to reduce your blood pressure in one of two ways. If your chiropractor is concentrating on your neck area, it's likely that he or she is helping to balance the activity of the sympathetic and parasympathetic nervous systems on the function of the heart and blood vessels. The mid-back area, on the other hand, is connected to kidney function; it is likely that your kidneys are producing more urine or the adrenal glands, which sit atop the kidneys, are producing a hormone that helps to lower blood pressure.

Q. What kind of training does a chiropractor usually have?

A. To be certified as a chiropractor, an individual studies at a chiropractic college for a minimum of four years. Training includes all of the basic science and diagnostic skills taught to a medical student, but does not involve surgical or pharmaceutical study. Some chiropractors also learn the fundamentals of nutrition.

Healing Touch: Bodywork and Massage

Q. After an unpleasant experience with Rolfing, which I found too painful, I've been hesitant to try other bodywork techniques. At the same time, I know that my posture is out of kilter, which is part of the reason I suffer from so much pain in my hips and knees. Is there another program that might help me?

A. Although Rolfing can be quite effective, it is not a painless method of manipulating the spine and joints. Many people with arthritis enjoy the slow, controlled, and gentle changes in posture that result from practicing the Alexander technique. Reread the section on this bodywork method in Chapter 10 and explore the resource section on page 168 for more information.

Q. Much to my surprise, my arthritis in my elbows, wrists, and fingers was greatly relieved by a massage therapist who concentrated, not on my arms, but on my feet. What's the connection?

A. It sounds as if your therapist is familiar with the concept of "reflexology," a form of massage in which the rest of the body is "projected" onto the foot. Remember, your body works as a unit, and whenever one part of it is injured, another part may well be affected. By massaging your feet, your therapist is helping to heal injured tissue in your feet that may have been referring pain to your arms for years.

The Power of Herbs

Q. I'm interested in treating my arthritis with herbs. But I also take medication for an ulcer. Can herbs interfere with the drugs I'm taking?

A. Herbs *are* drugs, and yes, if your physician and herbalist do not work together—or are at least aware of how each is treating you—you could run into some problems with the effectiveness of your treatment plan. It's up to you to supply all the people who treat you with a list of any and all medications and remedies you are taking.

Q. Is aromatherapy only used for relaxation or do the herbs from which oils are derived have physical effects as well?

A. First of all, it's important to realize that relaxation *is* physical. Remember, more and more evidence is surfacing every day that emotion, and thus the effects of emotion, are present in every cell of the body, including those of our muscles, tendons, ligaments, and bone. Second, there is some evidence that therapeutic particles of the original plants enter the body through the nasal passages and the skin and work internally the same way as a dose of herbal medicine by mouth would work.

Q. I'm allergic to penicillin and a variety of antibiotics. Could I be allergic to herbal remedies as well?

A. Absolutely, and you must be sure to inform your herbalist of any and all allergies and sensitivities to drugs and other substances you may have. This information will help him or her provide you with a safe, effective herbal remedy.

Like Cures Like: Homeopathy

Q. I visited a homeopath for the first time last week. After asking me lots of questions about my diet and other health problems, he decided to treat my arthritis with *Rhus tox*. I understand that this herb comes from the poison ivy plant. I'm quite allergic to poison ivy. Is this dangerous for me?

A. The amount of toxic substance in the homeopathic solution is quite minuscule and thus unlikely to provoke a serious allergic reaction. However, please make sure that the homeopath is aware of your allergy and keep close watch on your symptoms and side effects.

Q. I'm not sure I understand the way homeopathy works, and what I do know makes me unsure that it really does work, but I have friends who swear by it. Do I have to believe in it for the therapy to work?

A. Having faith that a treatment has the potential to work is certainly helpful, but it is not necessary for you to fully understand homeopathy to reap its benefits. In fact, many homeopaths are unsure themselves exactly how a substance diluted so many times still has the power to heal. Nevertheless, millions of people around the world find relief from a variety of ailments with homeopathy and you may be able to do so as well.

In the next section, we describe some of the vast resources available to you in your quest for a safer, more effective, and longer-lasting approach to relieving your back pain and bringing your whole body and spirit into a more balanced state.

Natural Resources

....

$\mathcal{M}$ore and more Americans are exploring the world of alternative medicine every day, and every day more and more resources become available to answer their questions and meet their growing need for quality health care.

Following are associations that provide information—lists of qualified professionals, pamphlets, videos to explain treatment philosophy, and other supportive material—about each type of alternative approach addressed in this book.

In addition, we also provide a brief bibliography listing some of the many books you can read in order to deepen your interest in and knowledge about alternative medicine.

Acupuncture/Chinese Medicine

American Academy of Medical Acupuncture
(for medical doctors who are acupuncturists)
5870 Wilshire Boulevard
Los Angeles, CA 90036
800-521-AAMA

National Oriental Medicine and Acupuncture Alliance (non-
M.D. acupuncturists)
638 Prospect Avenue
Hartford, CT 06195
203-232-4825

National Commission for the Certification of Acupuncturists
1424 16th St. NW
Washington, DC 20036
202-232-1404

READING LIST

Beinfeld, Harriet, and Korngold, Efrem. *Between Heaven and Earth: Guide to Chinese Medicine*. New York: Ballantine Books, 1991.

Kaptchuk, Ted. *The Web That Has No Weaver: Understanding Chinese Medicine*. New York: Congdon and Weed, 1992.

Reid, Daniel. *The Complete Book of Chinese Health and Healing*. Boston: Shambala, 1994.

Aromatherapy

Aromatherapy Institute of Research
P.O. Box 2354
Fair Oaks, CA 95628
916-965-7546

National Association for Holistic Aromatherapy
P.O. Box 17622
Boulder, CO 80308
303-258-3791

READING LIST

Hymann, Daniele. *Aromatherapy: The Complete Guide to Plant and Flower Essences*. New York: Bantam Books, 1991.

Lavabre, Marcel. *Aromatherapy Workbook*. Rochester, VT: Healing Arts Press, 1990.

Rose, Jeanne. *The Aromatherapy Book*. Berkeley, CA: North Atlantic Books, 1992.

Arthritis

American College of Rheumatology
60 Executive Park Drive South, Suite 150
Atlanta, GA 30329
(404) 633-3777

Arthritis Foundation
1314 Spring Street, NW
Atlanta, GA 30309
(404) 872-7100 (in Atlanta)
(800) 283-7800

The National Institute of Arthritis and Musculoskeletal
    and Skin Diseases
9000 Rockville Pike, Building 31, Room 4C32
Bethesda, MD 20892
(301) 496-4353

The Rheumatoid Disease Foundation
5106 Old Harding Road
Franklin, TN 37064

READING LIST

Eades, Mary Dan, M.D. *If It Runs in Your Family: Arthritis.*
    New York: Bantam Books, 1992.

Kantrowicz, Fred, M.D. *Taking Care of Arthritis.* New York:
    Harper-Perennial, 1991.

Lorrig, Kale, and Fries, James. *The Arthritis Helpbook.* Reading,
    MA: Addison-Wesley Publishing Co., 1990.

Murray, Michael T. *Arthritis: Getting Well Naturally.* Rocklin,
    CA: Prima Publishing, 1994.

Pisetsky, David, S., M.D., Ph.D., and Trien, Susan Flamholtz.
    The Duke University Medical Center Book of Arthritis.
    New York: Ballantine Books, 1992.

Ayurvedic Medicine

Ayurvedic Institute–Dr. Vasant Lad
11311 Menaul NE Suite A
Albuquerque, NM 87112
(505)291-9698

Ayurvedic Rehabilitation Center–Loretta Levitz
103 Bennett Street
Brighton, MA 02135
617-782-1727

American School of Ayurvedic Sciences
10025 NE 4th Street
Bellevue, WA 98004
206-453-8022

The College of Maharishi
Ayurveda Health Center
P.O. Box 282
Fairfield, IO 5256
515-472-5866

READING LIST

Chopra, Deepak, M.D. *Ageless Body, Timeless Mind.*
New York: Harmony Books, 1993. *Perfect Health*, 1991.
Quantum Healing, 1990.

Frawley, David, O.M.D. *Ayurvedic Healing.* Salt Lake City:
Morson Publishing, 1990.

Lad, Vasant. *Ayurveda: The Science of Self-Healing.* Santa Fe:
Lotus Press, 1988.

Biofeedback

Association for Applied Psychophysiology
  and Biofeedback Certification Institute of America
10200 West 44th Avenue, Suite 304
Wheat Ridge, CO 80033
303-422-8436

Center for Applied Psychophysiology
Menninger Clinic
P.O. Box 829
Topeka, KS 66601
913-273-7500

READING LIST

Danskin, David G., and Crow, Mark. *Biofeedback: An Introduction and Guide.* Palo Alto, CA: Mayfield Publishing Co., 1981.

Bodywork and Massage

American Massage Therapy Association
820 Davis Street, Suite 100
Evanston, IL 60201
708-864-0123

American Oriental Bodywork Therapy Association
6801 Jericho Turnpike
Syosset, NY 11791
516-364-5533

The Rolf Institute
205 Canyon Boulevard
Boulder, CO 80302
800-530-8875

North American Society of Teachers of the
    Alexander Techinique
P.O. Box 112484
Tacoma, WA 98411
800-473-0620

Zero Balancing Association
P.O. Box 1727
Capitola, CA 95010
408-476-0665

READING LIST

Benjamin, Ben E., Ph.D., and Borden, Gale, M.D. *Listen to Your Pain*. New York: Penguin Books, 1984

Smith, Fritz. *Inner Bridges*. Atlanta: Humanics, Ltd., 1994

Chiropractic and Osteopathy

American Chiropractic Association
1701 Clarendon Boulevard
Arlington, VA 22209
703-276-8800

Cranial Academy
3500 DePauw Boulevard
Indianapolis, IN 46268

International Chiropractors Association
1110 North Glebe Road, Suite 1000
Arlington, VA 22201
800-423-4690

World Chiropractic Alliance
2950 N. Dobson Road, Suite 1
Chandler, AZ 85224
800-347-1011

READING LIST

Coplan-Griffiths, Michael. *Dynamic Chiropractic Today: The
Complete and Authoritative Guide to This Major Therapy.*
San Francisco: Harper Collins, 1991.

Palmer, Daniel David. *The Chiropractor's Adjuster.* Davenport,
IA: Palmer College Press, 1992.

Diet and Nutrition

American College of Nutrition
722 Robert E. Lee Drive
Wilmington, NC 28480

American College of Advancement in Medicine
P.O. Box 3427
Laguna Hills, CA 92654
714-583-7666

READING LIST

Braverman, Eric R., M.D., and Pfeiffer, Carl C., M.D.
    The Healing Nutrients Within. New Canaan, CT:
    Keats Publishing, Inc., 1987.

Hass, Elson M., M.D. *Staying Healthy with Nutrition*. Berkeley,
    CA: Celestial Arts Publishing, 1992.

Herbal Medicine

The American Herbalists Guild
P.O. Box 1683
Soquel, CA 95073
408-438-1700

The American Botanical Council
P.O. Box 201660
Austin, TX 78720-1660
512-331-8868

Herb Research Foundation
1007 Pearl Street, Suite 200
Boulder, CO 80302
303-449-2265

The Natural Apothecary
167 Massachusetts Avenue
Arlington, MA 02174
617-641-1378

READING LIST

Castleman, Michael. *The Healing Herbs*. Emmaus, PA:
Rodale Press, 1991.

Hoffman, David. *The Herbal Handbook*. Rochester, VT:
Healing Arts Press, 1987.

Homeopathy

International Foundation for Homeopathy
2366 Eastlake Avenue
Seattle, WA 98102
206-324-8230

National Center for Homeopathy
801 North Fairfax
Alexandria, VA 22314
703-548-7790

American Institute of Homeopathy
1585 Glencoe
Denver, CO 80220
303-898-5477

READING LIST

Cummings, Stephen, M.D. *Everybody's Guide to Homeopathic Medicines*. Los Angeles: Jeremy P. Tarcher, Inc., 1991.

Lockie, Andrew. *The Family Guide to Homeopathy*. New York: Prentice Hall Press, 1993.

Ullman, Dana. *Discovering Homeopathy: Medicine for the 21st Century*. North Atlantic Books, 1991.

Meditation and Mind/Body Medicine

Institute of Transpersonal Psychology
P.O. Box 4437
Stanford, CA 94305
415-327-2066

Mind-Body Clinic
New England Deaconess Hospital
Harvard Medical School
185 Pilgrim Road
Cambridge, MA 02215
617-632-9530

Stress Reduction Clinic
University of Massachusetts Medical Center
55 Lake Avenue, North
Worcester, MA 01655
508-856-2656

The Center for Mind-Body Studies
5225 Connecticut Avenue NW
Washington, DC 20015
202-966-7388

READING LIST

Benson, Herbert. *The Relaxation Response.* New York: Outlet Books, Inc., 1993.

Borysenko, Joan. *Mending the Body, Mending the Mind.* New York: Bantam Books, 1988.

Locke, Steven, and Colligan, Douglas. *The Healer Within.* New York: Mentor, 1986.

Moyers, Bill. *Healing and the Mind.* New York: Doubleday, 1993.

Yoga

Himalayan Institute of Yoga, Science, and Philosophy
RRI Box 400
Honesdale, PA 18431
800-822-4547

International Association of Yoga Therapists
109 Hillside Avenue
Mill Valley, CA 94941
415-383-4587

READING LIST

Cummings, Stephen, M.D., and Ullman, Dana, M.P.H.
Everybody's Guide to Homeopathic Medicines. Los Angeles:
Jeremy P. Tarcher, Inc., 1991.

Hewitt, James. *The Complete Yoga Book.* New York:
Schocken Books, 1977.

Ullman, Dana. *Discovering Homeopathy: Your Introduction to
the Science and Art of Homeopathic Medicine.* Berkeley,
CA: North Atlantic Books, 1991.

Alternative Medicine/General Reading

American Association of Naturopathic Physicians
2366 Eastlake Avenue, Suite 322
Seattle, WA 98102
206-323-7610

American Holistic Medical Association
4101 Lake Boone Trail, Suite 201
Raleigh, NC 27607
919-787-5146

READING LIST

Goldberg Group (350 physicians). *Alternative Medicine: The Definitive Guide*. Puyallap, WA: Future Medicine Publishing, Inc., 1993.

Monte, Tom, and editors of "EastWest Natural Health." *WorldMedicine: The EastWest Guide to Healing Your Body*. New York: Tarcher/Perigree, 1993.

Murray, Michael, and Pizzorno, Joseph. *Encyclopedia of Natural Medicine*. Rocklin, CA: Prima Publishing, 1991.

Words and Terms to Remember

....

Active movement: Normal range of voluntary movement of a joint.

Acupoints: Acupuncture points throughout the body which correspond to specific organs.

Acupressure: A healing art based on the fundamentals of Chinese medicine in which finger pressure is applied to specific sensitive points on the body.

Acupuncture: A technique used in Chinese medicine that involves the insertion of small needles under the skin to activate the flow of energy within the body.

Aerobic exercise: Physical exercise that relies on oxygen for energy production.

Alexander technique: A technique concerned with improving posture to reduce or prevent arthritis.

Allopathy: Term for standard Western medicine; from the Greek *allos* (different) and *pathein* (disease, suffering) and thus implying the use of drugs whose effects are different from those of the disease being treated.

Anaerobic exercise: Exercise that draws upon the muscles' own stores of energy and does not require oxygen, such as weight-lifting and isometric exercises.

Analgesic: A drug that relieves pain, including aspirin, acetaminophen (Tylenol), Darvon, and codeine.

Ankylosing spondylitis: Disease characterized by lower back pain that spreads to the hips, knees, and heels; may be accompanied by fever, loss of appetite, and heart and lung problems; may cause spinal bones to fuse, causing the back to become rigid.

Antibodies: Protein substances produced by immune system cells that interact with and destroy cells or microbes perceived to be foreign to the body.

Antigens: Substances foreign or perceived to be foreign in the body; result in the production of antibodies.

Anti-inflammatory: Drugs designed to reduce swelling, inflammation, and pain. Some common antiinflammatory drugs include Feldene (piroxicam), Motrin (ibuprofen), and Voltaren (diclofenac sodium).

Arthritis: Inflammation and irritation of the joints; Greek for "swollen joint"; involves inflammation and/or pain of a joint or joints; may result in changes in the afflicted body part.

Arthroplasty: A surgical procedure involving joint reconstruction using the patient's own tissues as well as artificial joint components.

Arthroscopy: Examination of the inside of a joint through a slender, fiber optic instrument inserted through a small incision.

Articulation: The place of union, or junction, between two bones.

Autoimmune disease: Disease in which the immune system produces antibodies against the body's own cells, destroying healthy tissue.

Autonomic nervous system: The part of the nervous system responsible for bodily functions such as the heartbeat, blood pressure, and digestion. It is divided into two divisions, the sympathetic nervous system and the parasympathetic nervous system.

Biofeedback: A behavior modification therapy in which people are taught to control bodily functions such as blood pressure through conscious effort.

Bursa: A fluid-filled sac that forms a buffer between bones and tendons or ligaments; it is lined with a membrane that releases fluid and permits muscles, tendons, and bones to slide over each other.

Carbohydrates: Organic compounds of carbon, hydrogen, and oxygen, which include starches, cellulose, and sugars, and are an important source of energy. All carbohydrates are eventually broken down in the body to glucose, a simple sugar.

Cartilage: Rubbery material found at the end of each bone that absorbs shock and allows bones to move smoothly.

Central nervous system: The brain and the spinal cord, which are responsible for the integration of all neurological functions.

Channels: Also called *meridians*; in traditional Chinese medicine, the invisible pathways of life energy on the surface of and within the body.

Chinese medicine: A philosophy and methodology of health and medicine developed in ancient China.

Collagen: White, fibrous protein providing the framework for skin, tendons, bones, cartilage, and all other connective tissue.

Connective tissue: Highly vascular tissue that forms the supporting and connecting structure of the body; fascia is an example of connective tissue.

Contracture: A joint deformity caused by loss of joint movement and shortening of surrounding tissues.

Corticosteriods: Hormones produced in the cortex of the adrenal glands; drug versions of these hormones are used to treat inflammation.

CT scan: A computerized tomogram (x-ray image), reconstituted by a computer to depict bone and soft tissues in several planes.

Deficient condition: In traditional Chinese medicine, a disorder resulting from the body's inability to maintain equilibrium.

Detoxification: In Ayurveda, the process of removing toxins from the body.

Doshas: In Ayurvedic medicine, the three basic body types that determine an individual's constitution.

Endorphins: Natural substances produced by the body that function as natural painkillers.

Epinephrine: Also called adrenaline. A hormone secreted by the adrenal glands that increases the heart rate and constricts blood vessels.

Essential oil: Concentrated, pure aromatic essence extracted from plants.

Excess condition: In traditional Chinese medicine, a condition in which life energy (qi), blood, or body fluid is disordered and accumulates in channels or elsewhere in the body.

Extension: The range of motion of a joint.

Fascia: A sheet or band of connective tissue that separates various muscles and organs within the body.

Fibrositis: A disease involving pain in muscles or joints with no clinical signs of inflammation; also known as *fibromyalgia*.

Fight-or-flight response: The body's response to perceived danger or stress, involving the release of hormones and subsequent rise in heart rate, blood pressure, and muscle tension.

Five Phases theory: In Chinese medicine, a way of looking at the body and the universe that explains the interaction between them.

Fracture: An injury to a bone in which the tissue of the bone is broken.

Gluteus: Muscle of the buttocks.

Gout: An acute form of arthritis beginning in the joints of the knee or foot and related to an excess of uric acid in the blood.

Hamstring: The large muscle located at the back of the thigh.

Heberden's nodes: Bony growths in the finger joints that are a sign of osteoarthritis.

Holistic: Pertaining to the whole body; treatment of disease by taking into consideration every part of the body to bring the internal environment into balance.

Homeopathic remedy: A remedy that produces a reaction in a person similar to the symptoms beting treated.

Inflammation: A reaction to injury or infection resulting in redness, heat, swelling, pain, and loss of function in the affected area.

Isometric exercise: Exercise in which pressure is exerted against an immovable object, thus building muscle while keeping joints stationary.

Jinglo: Chinese term for channels or meridians, the network of invisible pathways of life energy (qi) in the body.

Joint: The structure created where two bones come together.

Joint capsule: Fibrous capsule encasing joint contents, including the ends of bones and cartilage; also called the *synovial sac*.

Juvenile rheumatoid arthritis: Term used to describe several types of arthritis that can occur in childhood.

Kapha: An Ayurvedic body type.

Law of Similars: The principle that "like shall be cured by like" that forms the basis of homeopathy; the proper remedy for a patient's disease is that substance that is capable of producing, in a healthy person, symptoms similar to those from which the patient suffers.

Ligament: A strong, elastic band that holds a joint together, and that in the spine keeps vertebrae in place by supporting and strengthening discs and vertebral joints.

Limbic system: A group of brain structures that influences the endocrine and autonomic motor systems.

Lupus: Also called systemic lupus erythematosus; autoimmune disease that can affect any organ or system in the body.

Lyme disease: An infectious disease contracted from a bite from a tick carrying *Borrelia burgdorferi,* a spirochete.

Manipulation: Technique used in chiropractic therapy to adjust the spine, joints, and other tissue.

Meridian: In traditional Chinese medicine, one of the fourteen channels in the body through which the energy known as qi runs.

Mobilization: A technique of chiropractic therapy that gently increases the range of movement of a joint.

Moxa: Dried mugwort leaves used in traditional Chinese medicine, placed on the end of needles then lighted and held near an acupuncture point to warm and tonify life energy (qi).

Muscles: Elastic tissues that support the joint and allow the body to move.

Muscle spasms: Involuntarily contracted, painful muscles.

Musculoskeletal system: The muscles and bones considered as a whole.

Myelogram: A radiologic test in which the spinal cord, nerves roots, and surrounding space can be visualized.

Neurological deficit: Loss of reflexes and/or normal motor strength.

Neurotransmitters: Substances that transmit messages to, from, and within the brain and other body tissues.

Nicotine: The addictive chemical substance derived from tobacco that affects blood pressure and brain activity.

Norepinephrine: A hormone secreted by the adrenal gland as a reaction to the "fight-or-flight response" that raises blood pressure and acts to stimulate muscle contraction.

Obesity: The condition in which excess fat has accumulated in the body; usually considered to be 20 percent above the recommended weight for height and age.

Orthopedic surgeon: A physician who specializes in surgery of the muscles, bones, joints, and related structures.

Osteoarthritis: A form of arthritis in which normally spongy cartilage cracks and flakes; the most common form of arthritis, presumed to be caused by wear and tear (and possible misuse) of a joint over time.

Osteopathy: A branch of Western medicine that focuses primarily on the manipulation of the musculoskeletal system while taking a holistic approach to health.

Osteoporosis: A condition in which the bones of the body lose minerals and thus become weak and porous.

Palpation: Physical examination of the body using hands to feel for abnormalities.

Parasympathetic nervous system: The division of the nervous system that, when stimulated, slows heart rate, lowers blood pressure, and slows breathing.

Pelvic tilt: The body position in which the abdominal muscles are contracted and the buttocks tucked down and under the spine.

Pitta: An Ayurvedic body type.

Potency: The dilution of homeopathic remedies to increase their effectiveness, thus giving them their therapeutic value.

Qi: In traditional Chinese medicine, the life force or energy of the body and the universe, which circulates through the body's channels.

Qi stagnation: Any blockage of energy in the body that interrupts the body's natural functions or the healing process.

Quadriceps: The muscles located in the front of the thighs.

Range of motion: Normal range of movement for each joint, used to measure severity of arthritis; a term used to describe certain exercises.

Reiter's syndrome: Inflammation of joints following severe intestinal or urinary tract infections, although may occur with no evidence of infection.

Rheumatism: General term for a condition characterized by inflammation and pain in muscles and joints.

Rheumatoid arthritis: Autoimmune disease in which the joint is damaged and the synovial membrane thickens. May also affect the heart, blood vessels, nerves, and muscles.

Rheumatoid factor: Antibody found in large quantities in those with rheumatoid arthritis.

Rheumatologist: Physician who specializes in diagnosing and treating joint problems, arthritis.

Risk factor: A condition or behavior that increases one's likelihood of developing a disease or injury.

Rolfing: A massage technique that focuses on realigning the fascia—the connective tissue that envelops the muscles and organs. The goal of Rolfing is structural integrity, or making sure that all of the organs, bones, and tissues are properly positioned within the body.

Shen: In traditional Chinese medicine, the "spirit" or consciousness, which both originates and forms the outward expression of human life.

Shiatsu: A massage technique developed in Japan and based on the Chinese medical theory that disease and pain are caused by blocked qi (energy) along energy pathways in the body. By applying pressure to the blocked meridian, relief from pain and disease may result.

Stress: Any factor, physical or emotional, that threatens the health of the body or otherwise requires a response or change.

Subluxation: In chiropractic, a term used to explain a misalignment of spinal vertebrae.

Succussion: The forceful shaking of liquid homeopathic remedies that allows the permeation of the original substance into the liquid medium.

Sympathetic nervous system: The division of the autonomic nervous system responsible for such actions as blood pressure, salivation, and digestion; works in balance with the parasympathetic nervous system.

Symptoms: Observable or internal changes in the mental, emotional, and physical condition of a person; in holistic medicine, symptoms are the external proof of an internal imbalance.

Synovial fluid: Clear, viscous fluid produced by the synovial membrane which acts as a joint lubricant.

Tao: The course of nature and ways of nature; a Chinese term denoting the universe as an undifferentiated whole.

Tendon: The connective fibers attaching the muscles to bones; when a muscle contracts, or shortens, it pulls on the tendon, which moves the bone.

Tendonitis: Inflammation of a tendon.

Tincture: An alcoholic solution of a medicinal substance.

Tonify: In Chinese medicine, to nourish, augment, and invigorate; to add to the supply of life energy (qi) and to promote the proper functioning and balance in the body.

Toxin: Substance that is harmful or poisonous to the body.

Trapezius: Muscle of the upper back.

Trigger points: Certain places on muscles that appear exceptionally tender to touch.

Vata: An Ayurvedic body type.

Vital force: In homeopathy, the intangible energy that animates all living creatures and mediates their physical, emotional, and intellectual responses to external stress.

Yang organs: In Chinese medicine, the yang organs are hollow or surface organs such as the large intestines, stomach, and gall-bladder.

Yin organs: In Chinese medicine, the yin organs are dense, internal organs such as the heart, liver, lungs, kidneys, and bones.

Yin/Yang: Chinese concept that describes all existence in terms of states or conditions that are different but mutually dependent; traditional Chinese medicine aims to restore balance to these contrasting aspects of the body and mind.

Index

About the Authors

....

Glenn S. Rothfeld, M.D.

Glenn S. Rothfeld, M.D., is founder and Medical Director of Spectrum Medical Arts in Arlington, Massachusetts, a comprehensive primary care center blending orthodox and complementary medical styles. He holds one of the nation's first Master's Degrees in acupuncture, and is director of Western Medical Curriculum at the New England School of Acupuncture. He is also Clinical Instructor at Tufts University School of Medicine, where he teaches a popular course in Natural Medicine.

Suzanne LeVert

Suzanne LeVert is a writer who specializes in health and medical subjects. Her recent titles include A Woman Doctor's Guide to Menopause, Parkinson's Disease: A Complete Guide for Patients and Caregivers, *and* If It Runs in the Family: Hypertension and Diabetes. *She lives in Boston, Massachusetts.*